NUTRITION UPDATE

NUTRITION UPDATE

Volume 2

Edited by

JEAN WEININGER, Ph.D.

GEORGE M. BRIGGS, Ph.D.

Department of Nutritional Sciences
University of California, Berkeley

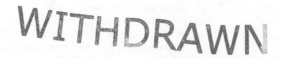

A Wiley-Interscience Publication
JOHN WILEY & SONS
New York • Chichester • Brisbane • Toronto • Singapore

Library of Congress Cataloging in Publication Data:

Main entry under title:

Nutrition update.

  "A Wiley-Interscience publication."
  Includes bibliographical references and index.
  1. Nutrition disorders. 2. Nutrition. 3. Nutrition
policy—United States. I. Weininger, Jean. II. Briggs,
George M. (George McSpadden), 1919–   [DNIM:
1. Nutrition. QU 145 N976]
RC620.N85 1985   613.2   82-20085
ISBN 0-471-09605-9

Printed in the United States of America

10 9 8 7 6 5 4 3 2 1

Series Preface

It is our intention that the *Nutrition Update* series will greatly assist people with diverse backgrounds and interests to keep informed about the latest breakthroughs, developments, and controversies in the fast moving field of human nutrition.

Nutrition Update is written primarily for nutrition educators, dietitians, college teachers of nutrition and related fields, public health nutritionists, and nutrition students at all levels. In addition, the subjects are chosen to be of interest to all types of health professionals and practitioners (including nurses, physicians, dentists, and public health workers), home economists, food scientists and technologists, health and science writers, and nutritionists working in academic institutions, industry, governmental agencies, agricultural extension, and other areas.

For the most part, *Nutrition Update* is written with a minimum of scientific jargon; its language is readily understood. Therefore, we feel it will also be valuable for large numbers of lay people who have an interest in their own nutrition and health and who want to keep up with new discoveries. Nutrition educators can recommend this series to those lay people who are looking for readable sources of reliable nutrition information.

This series is an outgrowth of an annual summary of current nutrition information that we started in 1974 as "Nutrition Update" articles for the *Journal of Nutrition Education*. That series continued until 1979. From the feedback we learned of the real need for a regular update of current nutrition developments in one volume, written so that it can be understood by and be useful to scientists and nonscientists. It is our regular practice to cover almost all of the world's nutrition literature in the original journals—updating, building up extensive files, and looking for topics and authors for *Nutrition Update*.

We have asked well-qualified scientists and professionals to bring us up to date in their field of expertise, to explore new ideas and controversies, to give their interpretation of the facts, and to provide practical dietary advice wherever possible. Many of our contributors are internationally known; some

v

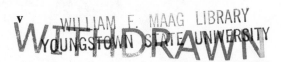

are younger people with new approaches in their field. All of them have excellent credentials and the respect of their colleagues. Each chapter is written specifically for *Nutrition Update*. These are not papers given at a symposium and then put together in a book.

In addition to serving as a reference book, each volume can serve as a textbook in courses on current issues and as supplementary reading material for undergraduate and graduate students in nutrition courses, and for students of medicine, nursing, and related health areas.

As the science of nutrition evolves, we intend to bring to the readers of this series researchers and thinkers who are on the leading edge of nutrition and who will address difficult questions: Where do we stand in nutrition today? What really matters in nutrition today? How can the results of nutrition research be translated into action in a way that contributes to the health, well-being, and quality of life of people all over the world?

Taken as a whole, we hope that these volumes will be a valuable record of the history of nutrition and, even more important, will help to point out how much we do *not* know and what remains to be discovered.

JEAN WEININGER
GEORGE M. BRIGGS

Preface

This second volume of the *Nutrition Update* series explores further some of the most important research and concerns in nutrition today. Illustrating the diversity which characterizes the field of nutrition, there is a potpourri of styles and approaches, as in the first volume. All of the authors are well qualified to present the latest information in their field. Many of them are internationally recognized for their expertise.

The topics covered in this volume complement those in *Nutrition Update*, Volume 1. Although no topic is repeated here, several of the chapters delve further into important issues raised in Volume 1. Taken together, and expanded by future volumes, the *Nutrition Update* series should provide a comprehensive update of the entire field of human nutrition.

We have grouped the chapters in this volume into five sections:

1. By featuring the section "Nutrition in Health and Disease," we are recognizing that many recent discoveries in nutrition are being applied in the health area, particularly with an eye toward prevention. Charles and Lorelei DiSogra, authors of the popular booklet *Nutrition and Cancer Prevention: A Guide to Food Choices*, write on current scientific thinking about nutrition and cancer prevention and the rationale behind emerging dietary recommendations. The well-known Canadian researcher Kenneth Carroll analyzes the relationship of dietary fat to breast cancer. Blending medical and dietetic perspectives, James Anderson and Beverly Sieling present nutritional guidance in the successful management of diabetes, including controversial new research about carbohydrates. The capabilities and limitations of nutritional treatment approaches, both prenatal and postnatal, to inherited metabolic disorders are discussed by Margaret Wallen and Seymour Packman. An essay by David Kritchevsky on the variability of serum cholesterol levels underscores how cautious we need to be before drawing conclusions, diagnosing disease, or assessing treatment based on a single laboratory test.

2. In the last volume, we looked at zinc, selenium, and dietary fiber in the "Nutrient Update" section. In this volume, Forrest Nielsen, one of the world's leading authorities on trace elements from the U.S.D.A.'s Grand Forks Human Nutrition Research Center, discusses the experimental evi-

dence for the essentiality of arsenic, nickel, silicon, and other "ultratrace" elements. This is a controversial area where there are great technical difficulties. Dr. Nielsen does an excellent job in revealing where we stand today with regard to these unusual nutrients.

3. The section "Special Foods and Diets" has a very practical focus. Experts from Loma Linda University discuss sound nutritional principles, and possible health benefits, for those wishing to follow various types of vegetarian diets. Harriet Kuhnlein brings much field experience in the United States and Canada to bear in her presentation of the potential nutrition contribution of wild plant and animal species to modern diets.

4. "Cultural Nutrition" provides new frames of reference with which to examine some important nutrition issues. Anthropologist Margaret Mackenzie looks at anorexia nervosa, bulimia, obesity, and the "fear of fatness" which is so prevalent in contemporary affluent societies. Basic research and policy implications are discussed in two critical areas. First, Sarah Samuels analyzes social and cultural factors that influence women in the United States to stop breastfeeding in the early postpartum period; and second, Barbara Underwood discusses the reproductive consequences of improved maternal nutrition in the preindustrialized world, considered in the context of the World Health Organization's goal of "health for all" by the end of the century.

5. Finally, "Nutrition Education" is discussed by two nutrition educators with much experience and expertise. Helen Ullrich reviews advances in accessibility and effectiveness of nutrition education programs during the last decade. Audrey Tittle Cross looks at the possibilities of using television as a positive contribution to nutrition education.

Among those topics we expect to include in the next volume are: nutrition and aging; weight-reducing diets; nutrition and brain chemistry; hair analysis for nutrition assessment; computers in nutrition education; food for athletic performance; nutrition in medical schools; world hunger issues; behavior and nutrition; vitamin D; dental health; the astronauts' diet; drug-nutrient interactions; methodology in public health nutrition; and an analysis of the scientific nutrition literature available today.

Please feel free to write to either of the editors with your constructive evaluation of any of the chapters or with your suggestions about future topics.

JEAN WEININGER
GEORGE M. BRIGGS

Department of Nutritional Sciences
University of California
Berkeley, California 94720

January 1985

Acknowledgments

Among those many people who have contributed to this second volume of the *Nutrition Update* series, we would like to thank the following, in particular: Henry Mooney, Jane-Ellen Long, and Sally Wells, for producing camera-ready copy from the manuscript; Dominic Federico, Ellen Satrom, Stewart Esposito, and Ben Weininger, for personal support, encouragement, and inspiration; and the 20 people who persevered through the undoubtedly difficult experience of writing a chapter in a multi-authored book.

Contents

Contents of Volume 1

SECTION THREE   NUTRITION IN THE LIFE CYCLE

SECTION FOUR   NUTRITION POLICY AND FOOD ADVERTISING

NUTRITION UPDATE

Nutrition in Health and Disease

1

Nutrition and Cancer Prevention

A PERSPECTIVE ON DIETARY RECOMMENDATIONS

CHARLES A. DISOGRA, M.P.H.
School of Public Health
University of California, Berkeley

LORELEI K. DISOGRA, Ed.D., R.D.
Director, Wellness Program
Merritt Peralta Institute
Oakland, California

Address correspondence to Charles A. DiSogra, Dr.P.H. Candidate, Public Health Nutrition Program, 419 Warren Hall, School of Public Health, University of California, Berkeley, California 94720.

ABSTRACT

Nutrition is increasingly being recognized as playing a significant role in the cause and prevention of cancer. In 1984, both the American Cancer Society (ACS) and the National Cancer Institute (NCI) issued dietary recommendations to reduce the risk of cancer. The ACS and NCI dietary recommendations are rooted in the 1982 interim dietary guidelines to reduce cancer risk proposed by the National Academy of Sciences and are consistent with the well-known *Dietary Guidelines for Americans* (1980). Research on cancer risk now justifies prudent guidelines concerning dietary factors, such as fat, fiber, vitamins A and C, nitrites, cruciferous vegetables, charred foods, and alcohol. Recommendations to change the way most Americans eat have become a key component of NCI's prevention strategy. If the risk of various cancers could be reduced by changes in dietary patterns, an exciting potential for cancer prevention would exist.

One of the most important issues today in the area of public health nutrition is the relationship between diet and the cause of cancer. Increasing recognition of this relationship has recently culminated in the publication of dietary recommendations for cancer risk reduction. The concept that nutritional factors may play a role in the development of cancer is not new. What is new is that the accumulated evidence now supports a belief that changes in dietary patterns can reduce the risk of cancer. This belief is now embraced by leaders at the National Cancer Institute (NCI) and the American Cancer Society (ACS). Diet has become an important dimension of a national cancer prevention strategy. The resultant policy decisions have launched a broader direction for nutrition education and reinforce the concept that diet plays an important role in preventing chronic diseases.

The importance of a nutrition and cancer prevention relationship is emphasized further when the disease itself is put in perspective. It is estimated that cancer will claim 450,000 American lives in 1984. With the exception of heart disease, this is more than any other cause of death. Additionally, 870,000 new cancer cases are expected this year. It has also been estimated that the cost of medical care related to cancer will exceed 20 billion dollars in 1984 (1). Given these tremendous emotional and financial costs and the tragedy of lost lives, the prevention of cancer through all possible means is of utmost concern to public health professionals.

If the risk of various cancers can be reduced by changes in dietary patterns, an exciting potential exists to prevent a significant number of cancer cases from occurring. Although this concept has been around since the middle of the nineteenth century, the most convincing scientific data have only been produced during the past 20 years. With this accumulation of evidence, and an increased level of research activity, epidemiologists have been involved in what Ernst Wynder and Gio Gori have called the "epidemiological exercise" of quantifying the overall contribution of diet to cancer risk (2). Gori's own estimates in 1977 were that 30–40% of all cancers in men and 60% of all cancers in women were related to diet (3). In 1981, British epidemiologists Doll and Peto estimated that, for all cancers, 35% of the risk was attributed to diet (4). This estimate of diet's attributable risk varies greatly for different types of cancer. For example, they estimate that diet accounts for 90% of the risk for bowel cancer, 50% for breast cancer, 20% for lung cancer, and as little as 10% for some other cancers. Admittedly, these percentages for individual cancer types are "guesstimates"; however, Doll and Peto's overall estimate of 35% is currently the most accepted and quoted figure.

In 1982 the National Academy of Sciences (NAS) released its pivotal report on diet, nutrition, and cancer (5). The report concluded that the American population will eventually have the option of adopting a diet that could reduce its incidence of cancer by approximately one-third. After a critical review of the current literature, the Academy proposed an interim set of dietary guidelines for cancer risk reduction. These guidelines suggested that diets high in fat, and containing few fresh fruits, vegetables, and whole grains increase the risk of certain types of cancer. Consumption of salt-cured and smoked foods, alcohol, naturally occurring mutagens and contaminants were also associated with increased risk.

The NAS guidelines confronted policy-makers with the challenge of what to do about implementation. There have been few widely accepted consensus statements for the public on diet and cancer from either government or voluntary agencies. Those persons who felt diet was a risk factor for cancer and wanted to do something about it were left largely to the self-serving information marketed by the health food industry. The NAS guidelines offered a hope that much of the confusion, misinformation, and some of the cancer fatalism could be dispelled. With the potential of doing the greatest good for the greatest number of people, an ethical imperative existed to promote guidelines for cancer risk reduction. The NAS guidelines are nutritionally sound and somewhat similar to the dietary guidelines promoted for the last 25 years to reduce the risk of heart disease.

Before reviewing the individual dietary components associated with cancer, it is important to understand the criteria behind the judgments about what recommendations to make. Rather than depending on any single study to provide the elusive conclusive evidence, the ideal judgment is based on the results of several different types of studies. These are: epidemiological studies; tests on experimental animals; *in vitro* tests for genetic toxicity; and clinical trials using nutrition interventions with high risk subjects.

A variety of epidemiological investigations provide information about the occurrence of cancer in people and the foods consumed by those people. In case-control studies, the diets of persons who have a specific cancer are compared with the diets of a control population of cancer-free persons. Other epidemiological studies look at the populations of different countries, regions, and cultural or religious groups to compare mortality rates for specific cancers with their respective dietary patterns. An important extension of this is the use of migration studies, examining the cancer incidence or mortality rates of people who move from one country to another. For example, in Japan there is a low rate of breast and colon cancer. However, among descendents of Japanese who have migrated to the United States, the rates of breast and colon cancer are similar to the higher American rates. A change to the high-fat American diet from the traditional low-fat diet in Japan is one of the prime suspects for this difference in cancer rates.

In addition to epidemiological studies, laboratory investigations provide the well-controlled experiments for testing hypotheses and exploring related biological mechanisms of function and causation. Rats and mice are the most commonly used laboratory animals for testing the effects of different diets on the development of cancer. Studies using bacteria or tissue cultures are also employed to identify substances that are carcinogens and/or mutagens.

Another type of investigation is the clinical trial in which persons at high risk for a specific cancer are placed on a diet hypothesized to lower that risk. After a number of years, the cancer rate of this experimental group is compared to a control group that was not on the special diet. Good examples are two nationwide clinical trials currently being carried out by the NCI. One involves women with known risk factors for breast cancer (e.g., family history); the other involves women who formerly had breast cancer. Both are five-year studies employing low fat diets where 20% of the total calories is from fat.

Concordance of findings from several of these types of studies allows some conclusions to be drawn about the role of dietary components in the development of cancer. Standards at the NCI ideally require that criteria of consistency, temporality, strength, specificity, and coherence be met when drawing conclusions about diet and cancer studies. Consistency means many studies with similar conclusions. Temporality requires that the observed relationship holds up over time, that is, trends in consumption and cancer incidence support the relationship. Strength refers to the magnitude of significant differences observed in findings. The absence of alternative hypotheses regarding observations is the criterion of specificity that should be satisfied. And finally, a biological plausibility, or coherence of explanatory biomechanisms, should exist. It is these criteria that uphold the current and prudent judgments about the role of diet in the development and prevention of cancer.

A key difficulty in conducting studies on what people eat is the less than perfect methodology for collecting dietary data. Obtaining information on what people are currently eating by record keeping, recall, or reporting the frequency of consumption of specific food items is well documented as being problematic (6–11). A concern in some cancer studies arises when persons are asked to recall their diet of some period 10 or 20 years ago. The reasoning that necessitates this is the belief that a particular dietary pattern over many years is what may have contributed to the presence or absence of a certain cancer. A number of factors, including the person's current condition (e.g., the presence of cancer or some other medical condition), may distort dietary recollection. Additionally, the beginning stages of a patient's disease at some time before diagnosis may have caused a change in the person's food choices. It is these types of uncertainties that cause many an investigator sleepless nights. In most cases, the methods employed are the most practical possible and are chosen because of the lack of a more precise alternative. In light of this, results must always be interpreted with caution and good judgment.

It should be noted that the data for almost all studies are site specific. For example, a study on diet and breast cancer is the usual type of investigation as opposed to a very general study of diet and "cancer". When one speaks of increasing or decreasing the risk of cancer by dietary manipulation, the data support those judgments for specific sites only. Generalizations to cover all cancers, or unstudied sites, should not be made without due caution, if made at all. Also, association is not the same as causation. For example, while it may be increasingly evident that high-fat diets are associated with breast cancer, it would be erroneous to state that dietary fat causes cancer. Issues of causation and the role of dietary components in the mechanisms of carcinogenesis will ultimately be settled by laboratory investigators. Such investigations to date have proposed hypotheses about a variety of naturally occurring carcinogens and mutagens as well as anticarcinogens and antimutagens (12).

DIETARY FACTORS AND RISK OF CANCER

Dietary Fat

Excessive dietary fat has been linked to an increased risk for cancer of the breast, colon, prostate, testes, endometrium, and ovary. Evidence for this relationship shows the greatest strength of association and consistency of findings of all studied dietary components. Although saturated and unsaturated fats have been examined separately in epidemiological studies and in various combinations in animal studies, it appears that total fat consumption is the real influencing factor. For more than a decade, several studies have demonstrated a high positive correlation between the intake of fat and breast cancer mortality rates (13–17). In fact, laboratory studies in the early 1940s showed dietary fat enhancing mammary tumors in mice (18). These findings have been consistent over the years. Although studies have convincingly demonstrated an increased risk for induced mammary tumors in rats fed high-polyunsaturated fat diets, the overall data support the general importance of *total* dietary fat as playing a cancer promotion role in tumor development (19,20). Case-control studies involving women with breast cancer have shown that high-fat diets increase the risk for this disease (21,22).

Although a variety of international and case-control studies have associated high-fat diets with cancer of the testes (15), endometrium (15,17), ovary (23), pancreas (24,25), and prostate (13,14,26,27), colon cancer has received the most study relating to dietary fat. The fact that colon cancer is second only to lung cancer as the cause of cancer deaths underlines the importance of this association.

Colon cancer is primarily a problem of Western industrialized countries whose diets can be broadly characterized as being both high in fat and low in fiber. Low-fiber diets have, therefore, also been associated with colon and rectal cancer. Thus it is strongly suspected that the risk for colon cancer, and to a lesser extent rectal cancer, may involve both of these dietary components.

When different countries are compared for their consumption of fat and mortality due to colon cancer, a strong positive association is observed (15). Some studies, including case-control studies, have suggested that saturated fat from meat consumption, particularly beef, may be the most important factor (28–30). However, a number of animal studies have suggested a promotional effect of bile acids on tumorigenesis (31,32). Increases in the consumption of dietary fat result in increased bile acid production. High concentrations of bile acids greatly enhance the appearance of tumors in animal colons subjected to known carcinogens (33–35).

All of this research strongly suggests that a reduction in total dietary fat intake would be a prudent recommendation. It has been estimated that the American population currently consumes either 36% or 41% of total calories from fat. The two different estimates are derived from the National Food Consumption Survey (NFCS), 1977–78, and the Second National Health and Nutrition Examination Survey (NHANES-II), 1976–80, respectively. Much of the difference between these two survey estimations is rooted in their methodologies (36). The true figure probably lies somewhere in the range of 36–41%. The U. S. Dietary Goals, issued in 1977, recommended a diet with 30% of the calories from fat (37). This has become the minimum recommendation for cancer risk reduction. However, NCI recommends a diet that is below 30% and perhaps closer to 20% for maximum benefit. For many Americans, achieving this NCI goal would mean cutting their dietary fat intake almost in half. Such low-fat diets are not known to be in any way injurious to health, and, as part of a balanced diet with adequate total calories, would reduce the risk for both cancer and heart disease.

Fiber

For more than a decade it has been hypothesized that dietary fiber, the indigestible carbohydrate components of plants, plays a role in protecting against colon cancer (38). Western industrialized countries with low-fiber diets have been observed to have high mortality rates due to colon cancer; however, those same diets are also high in fat. It is therefore difficult to separate the effect of fiber alone and attempts to do so have been inconclusive (39). Case-control studies have demonstrated an inverse relationship between dietary fiber and colon cancer (40–43). Some laboratory studies suggest a protective effect for bran and cellulose from chemically induced carcinogens in rats and mice (44,45). In human populations, it has been suggested that the pentosan fraction of whole wheat may be a specific fiber component offering some protection from colon cancer (46).

In addition to this limited but persuasive scientific evidence, much of fiber's popularity and support comes from the believable mechanisms proposed as possible roles for fiber in protecting the large bowel. First, the enormous water holding capacity of fiber, particularly fiber from vegetable sources, is believed to result in a dilution of carcinogens in fecal matter. Second, bulkier fecal matter, due to water-laden fiber, has a shorter transit time through the colon, thus minimizing mucosal exposure to carcinogens. Third, it is believed that the presence of fiber influences fecal flora and/or bile acids which would otherwise enhance or promote tumorigenesis.

In order to take advantage of any possible benefit to reduce the risk of colon cancer, a diet that contains whole wheat products and generous daily servings of fruits and vegetables would be recommended. Both ACS and NCI recommend an increase in the consumption of dietary fiber. With the average American now consuming 10–20 g of dietary fiber each day, NCI has recommended that this amount be increased to a range of 25–35 g/day. Increasing the proportion of fiber-containing foods while decreasing the proportion of meat, fats and oils would be the best preventive dietary strategy. Wise food choices should preclude the unnecessary expense of supplementing a diet with purified fiber products.

Vitamin A/β-Carotene

A great deal of research has accumulated supporting a possible cancer preventive role for vitamin A. Much of the epidemiological research has demonstrated an inverse relationship between the consumption of β-carotene-rich foods and several kinds of cancer. β-carotene is the precursor and plant form of vitamin A that is transformed to vitamin A in the body by enzymatic action. Preformed vitamin A, also known as retinol, exists in some animal products such as liver and milk.

The epidemiological evidence linking vitamin A with a lower cancer risk is strongest where vegetables containing β-carotene have been consumed. Case-control studies with lung cancer patients have shown a lower risk for this disease associated with a high consumption of β-carotene foods (47–50). Similar significant associations have demonstrated a lower risk for cancer of the bladder (51), colon–rectum (52), larynx (53), esophagus (54), stomach (55), and prostate (27).

Most of the laboratory experiments with mice and rats support the concept of vitamin A being a protective agent against cancer. Animals deficient in vitamin A, when exposed to known chemical carcinogens, developed more tumors (lung, urinary bladder, large bowel) than animals that were not deficient in vitamin A (56–58). Other studies with animals have shown that high levels of vitamin A have also had some protective effect against chemically induced cancers of the lung, respiratory tract, stomach, cervix, and skin (56,59,60). Because vitamin A at high dosages is toxic, some animal experiments have been conducted with retinoids. These are synthetic compounds that are similar but not identical to retinol (vitamin A) and are referred to as vitamin A analogues. These experiments have shown these analogues to be effective in preventing the initial phases of cancer development in the lung, urinary bladder, breast, and skin of laboratory animals (61,62).

It would make good sense to apply these promising research findings regarding vitamin A/β-carotene. A potential advantage can be obtained by increasing the consumption of foods that are considered good sources of vitamin A/β-carotene. The dark leafy green and the yellow-orange vegetables, and carotene-rich yellow-orange fruits (such as cantaloupe, apricots, or peaches) would be the preferred food choices. According to NCI and ACS cancer prevention recommendations, these foods should be part of a daily diet. The use of vitamin A supplements is not encouraged because high dosages taken over a long period of time can be toxic. The combination of vitamin A in foods and the vitamin supplement could unknowingly result in high doses. Also, all the epidemiological research associates vitamin A/β-carotene-rich *foods* and not supplements with a reduced cancer risk. Not enough is known, however, to assume that only the vitamin A is producing a benefit for humans. This is currently being investigated further with a large-scale randomized trial employing the β-carotene supplementation of male physician subjects (63). In any event, increasing consumption of fruits and vegetables will also add to the intake of beneficial fiber, other vitamins, and minerals.

Vitamin C

There is very limited epidemiological evidence concerning vitamin C; however, for the few studies that have been done, an inverse relationship was observed. A significant association has been reported between the consumption of fresh fruits known to be high in vitamin C and a low risk for cancer of the esophagus and stomach (64–67). One recent case-control study suggested a possible protective effect of vitamin C for laryngeal cancer (68), and another study suggested the same effect for the early development of cervical cancer (53).

Experimentation with laboratory animals using ascorbic acid (vitamin C) has not been very convincing. However, there are studies that suggest an inhibitory effect for high dosages of ascorbic acid on chemically induced cancer in rats, although in some cases the number of animals used in the experiments was small (69–71).

It has been well demonstrated that ascorbic acid does inhibit the formation of carcinogenic nitrosamines (72). This is currently the most convincing role for vitamin C in a diet to reduce cancer risk. Nitrates and nitrites, naturally present in vegetables but most notably added as a preservative in processed meats and other food products, will react with amines and amides to form nitrosamines. This reaction naturally occurs in the mouth and stomach; it also occurs when preserved meats are cooked. Ascorbic acid inhibits this reaction and for this reason is added to cured meat products such as bacon in the form of sodium erythrobate or sodium ascorbate. Mice fed nitrite and ascorbic acid were found to have fewer tumors than those without the ascorbic acid in their diet (72,73).

At this point, the evidence for reduced cancer risk would suggest some relationship to vitamin C. Findings do not justify taking large supplemental doses of vitamin C for prevention of cancer. The evidence for vitamin C does support a broad recommendation to include generous servings of fruits and vegetables in a diet designed to reduce cancer risk. Again, both ACS and NCI encourage the daily intake of foods rich in vitamin C. Vitamin C is water-soluble and easily destroyed by cooking. To preserve the maximum amount of vitamin C in cooked foods, any steaming, stir-frying or boiling should be done quickly and briefly.

Selenium

The mineral selenium has received much attention as having a possible protective effect against cancer. Although there is no case-control evidence, there have been some geographical correlation studies that demonstrated a reduced risk of cancer associated with increased levels of selenium intake (74–77). Experiments with selenium in the diets of mice and rats exposed to chemical or viral carcinogenic agents have, in most cases, shown a reduction in the number of resulting tumors (78–81). It is well understood that selenium is an essential component of the enzyme glutathione peroxidase, which is known to protect cells from oxidative damage caused by free radicals. This is the most plausible biological mechanism for selenium in protecting genetic material. However, the maximum level of enzyme activity is achieved at levels of dietary intake below what is considered normal in the American diet (82). Since there is an adequate amount of selenium available in foods such as whole grains, meat, and seafood, there is no evidence of any benefit to be derived from selenium supplements. Another good reason to avoid supplements is that toxic levels of selenium exist only slightly above the 50–250 μg range of safe and adequate intake as set by the Committee on Dietary Allowances (National Research Council). Since the evidence for selenium and cancer risk is relatively weak, no cancer prevention recommendations have been made.

Nonnutrient Inhibitors in Food

A number of nonnutrient chemical compounds existing in foods have been demonstrated to inhibit cancer in laboratory animals. One relatively promising group of compounds is referred to as the "indoles" (a name derived from their shared indole molecular structure). They are of interest because of the very suggestive epidemiological and laboratory data supporting the cancer inhibitory effect of indole-containing foods in humans and animals, and of the isolated indole compounds in animals. These indoles are commonly found in the cabbage (*Brassicaceae*) family of vegetables. This family, sometimes referred to as the cruciferous vegetables, consists of Brussels sprouts, cabbage, turnips, broccoli, and cauliflower. Case-control studies have shown a relationship between the consumption of these vegetables, particularly Brussels sprouts and cabbage, and a reduced risk for colon cancer (83,84).

Laboratory experiments have demonstrated that rodents on diets that included these cruciferous vegetables had significantly fewer mammary tumors and less forestomach cancer after being exposed to known chemical carcinogens including benzopyrene (83,84). The significance of benzopyrene is that this carcinogen is readily produced when foods are burned, charred, smoked or grilled. Therefore, it is commonly consumed and virtually unavoidable in most cooked foods. The proposed inhibitory mechanism is that indoles greatly increase the activity of aryl-hydrocarbon hydroxylase, a defensive enzyme system, which, in effect, "neutralizes" the carcinogenic benzopyrene-like compounds and allows the body to excrete them. Since it is a wise strategy to keep one's defenses up, it is now being recommended that cruciferous vegetables be included in the diet frequently.

Benzopyrene

Since the early 1960s it has been reported that polycyclic aromatic hydrocarbons, such as benzopyrene, are formed on the surface of foods that are grilled or charcoal-broiled. Most of these compounds are mutagenic, having caused inheritable genetic damage in bacteria. Some of these same mutagens are also carcinogens. One of these carcinogens is benzopyrene, which, in a purified form, is used in laboratory experiments to induce cancer in animals. Investigators have measured the amount of benzopyrene that is formed on the burned or charred surface of foods (85–87) or is permeated throughout foods that have been cured by a smoking process (88). Most of the initial work looked at charcoal-broiled or grilled meat and fish; however, benzopyrene has been found in many other cooked protein foods (89).

There have been no epidemiological studies attempting to investigate an association between smoke-cured foods, or the burned material of cooked foods, and cancer in humans. Despite this fact, the strength of the laboratory data has encouraged ACS to recommend moderation in the consumption of smoked foods. NCI makes the same recommendation plus goes further to recommend cooking methods which minimize the formation of benzopyrene and other mutagens on foods. These methods include grilling or frying at lower temperatures (below 300°F) and, when charcoal broiling, wrapping foods in foil to reduce contact with smoke and flame. The recommended alternative cooking methods for limiting benzopyrene intake are: baking, steaming, stewing, roasting, or microwave cooking without a char-producing browning plate.

Each summer, an occasional newspaper article raises public awareness about carcinogens and mutagens produced when barbecuing. If cancer prevention education is successful, perhaps the benefits of cabbage (as in coleslaw) and other cruciferous vegetables will get communicated at the same time. Using low-fat cuts of meat would be additional helpful advice.

Coffee

There have been few convincing case-control studies associating coffee consumption with cancer. The concern for a possible risk for pancreatic cancer due to coffee drinking was reported in 1981 (90). A similar increased risk was also associated with decaffeinated coffee (91). There is no experimental evidence to support these findings. Instant, regular, and decaffeinated coffee are all mutagenic, but caffeine itself is not a mutagen (92). Since the roasting of coffee creates polycyclic aromatic hydrocarbons including benzopyrene (88), this probably accounts for the mutagenic activity. Caffeine has not caused cancer in laboratory animals (93). It has been reported, however, that other constituents of coffee may act as catalysts for nitrosamine formation (94). It cannot be stated at this time that coffee consumption has any effect on cancer risk; therefore, no recommendations have been made.

Alcohol

The consumption of alcohol was reported as associated with cancer as early as 1910, in France. Since then a number of studies have implicated alcoholic beverages as increasing the risk for cancer of the mouth, throat, esophagus, and lung (95–99). One recent French study suggests an association between red wine and stomach cancer (100). An increased risk for colon and rectal cancer has been observed among beer drinkers (101). One new study estimates that men who consume 3.5 cans of beer a day have three times more chance for rectal cancer then do nondrinkers. Whiskey or wine consumption at 50 oz/month was estimated as doubling the risk for lung cancer (102).

Ethanol itself is not a carcinogen; therefore, many of the other chemicals that differentiate alcoholic beverages are suspect. The major concern is the synergistic relationship between alcohol and tobacco smoke. This interactive role between tobacco and alcohol greatly increases the risk for cancer of the mouth, larynx, and esophagus (97,103). It has also been suggested that this synergism increases the risk for respiratory tract cancers (104). All of these studies should spell caution for heavy consumers of alcohol, particularly drinkers who smoke. Also, the impaired nutritional status of heavy drinkers is an additional factor that may exacerbate cancer risk. The current recommendation is for moderation in the consumption of alcohol.

Obesity

A person is considered obese if he or she is 20% or more over ideal body weight. There are many factors that make studies of obesity and its relationship to cancer risk difficult to interpret. Some of these factors have to do with sorting out the effects of specific nutrients, such as dietary fat, from the overall caloric intake of obese persons. In one very large study, conducted by ACS, obesity had been associated with an increased incidence of cancers of the uterus, gallbladder, kidney, stomach, colon, and breast. Men and women 40% or more overweight were found to have a 33% and 55%, respectively, greater risk for cancer than persons of normal weight (105). The association of obesity with an increased risk for breast cancer is thought to be stronger for postmenopausal women than for premenopausal women (106,107).

Maintaining an ideal body weight to avoid obesity is a good recommendation, particularly for postmenopausal women. ACS is promoting a recommendation to avoid obesity in order to reduce cancer risk.

Other Dietary Factors

Several other dietary factors, notably vitamin E, food additives, B vitamins, nonnutrient food constituents that are mutagenic, aflatoxin, and a variety of other contaminants have been studied in an attempt to understand their relationship to human cancer risk. With the exceptions of aflatoxin and certain food additives, there has not been adequate research to draw any conclusions about these other dietary factors and cancer in humans.

Aflatoxins are produced by ubiquitous molds that grow on damp grains, nuts, and seeds. Aflatoxin B_1 is a powerful carcinogen known to cause liver cancer in rats (108). Few epidemiological studies have shown an aflatoxin association with liver cancer in humans; therefore, no conclusions about cancer risk have been drawn. Avoiding a known carcinogen, however, is always a good idea. Aflatoxin contamination of stored commodities poses more of a problem in tropical climates than in the North American food supply. The presence of other contaminants in the food supply raises important environmental issues that go beyond the scope of this paper. NCI recommends avoiding moldy nuts and seeds to minimize aflatoxin intake.

An exhaustive review of the scientific literature is available in the 1982 report by the NAS Committee on Diet, Nutrition, and Cancer (5). A second report by that same committee provides suggestive directions for future research (109). Recently, Willett and MacMahon have also examined epidemiological and laboratory data and hypotheses in a two-part diet and cancer overview (110,111).

THE EMERGENCE OF DIETARY RECOMMENDATIONS

Prior to 1981, dietary recommendations to reduce cancer risk were chiefly those written by individuals. The occasional, and usually overcautious, article in scientific journals tended to focus on the dietary component(s) of interest to the author and was not written as guidance for the public. The mass media, by default, became the primary guiding source for public information related to diet and cancer. Unfortunately, this did not always prove reliable or accurate. Research findings are too often reduced by the press to newsworthy headlines that overstate conclusions. Press reports generally present the results of one study and usually emphasize a single dietary component. Undoubtedly, this has caused both alarm and confusion among people concerned about a relationship between food and cancer. An unjustified belief persisted that just about everything caused cancer and that nothing could be done to avoid the disease. Such a fatalistic attitude defies informed preventive action. Since everyone has to eat, and some would like to take steps to reduce their risk of cancer, an environment existed that was ripe for charlatanism. Many individuals promoted their own prescription for diets to prevent cancer while the government and private agencies remained silent.

In light of this, one might have asked what the scientific community could reasonably tell the American public. With billions of dollars spent on cancer research, what had been learned about preventing cancer? Such a question, aimed at NCI, was raised by the U.S. Congress in the late 1970s. In 1980, NCI responded by requesting the National Academy of Sciences to appoint a special committee to review the literature, develop interim guidelines for the public, and provide recommendations for further research in the area of diet, nutrition, and cancer.

Also in 1980, ACS funded a small research project to produce and field test a prototype public education booklet on nutrition and cancer prevention. It is important to note that in 1980 ACS did not have a position or policy on diet and cancer. In 1981, the project successfully produced a 28-page consumer booklet entitled *Nutrition and Cancer Prevention: A Guide to Food Choices* (112). This booklet made specific nutrition recommendations to reduce the risk of cancer. These recommendations were, in substance, similar to the NAS interim guidelines released the following year. Despite very limited project publicity, and no publicity by the ACS organization (the booklet was not considered an official ACS publication), over 250,000 booklets were requested from 1981 to 1983. Besides demonstrating public interest, this project illustrated that scientific information on nutrition and cancer prevention could be successfully translated and packaged for the public.

In 1982, the NAS released its report, *Diet, Nutrition, and Cancer*, that included interim dietary guidelines for the public to reduce cancer risk (5). Although they specified their guidelines as "interim," the committee concluded that there was sufficient justification for guidelines to be issued. NCI accepted this report and soon initiated plans to act on the report's findings.

In early 1984, NCI launched a major new cancer prevention awareness program targeting health professionals and the public. Dietary modification had now become a legitimate strategy within NCI's **cancer control activities to achieve their overall goal of reducing the**

NUTRITION UPDATE

Table 1. A Summary and Comparison of Cancer Risk Reduction Dietary Recommendations Issued by the National Academy of Sciences (NAS), the National Cancer Institute (NCI), and the American Cancer Society (ACS)

Risk Factor	Agency (Year)		
	NAS (1982)	NCI (1984)	ACS (1984)
Total fat (% of calories)	Reduce to 30%	Reduce to 30% or below	Reduce to 30%
Fiber (vegetables, fruit, whole grains)	Daily	Increase to 25-35 g/day (several servings per day)	Eat more
Vitamin A/ β-carotene foods	Frequently	Daily	Daily
Vitamin C foods	Frequently	Daily	Daily
Cruciferous vegetables (indoles)	Frequently	Several servings per week	Include in diet
Charred or smoked foods (benzopyrene)	Minimize	Choose less often	Moderation in smoked foods only
Alcohol	Moderation	Moderation	Moderation
Nitrites (cured/ preserved foods)	Minimize	-	Moderation
Supplements (vitamins, etc.)	No	No	No
Selenium	-	-	-
Aflatoxins	-	Avoid	-
Obesity	-	-	Avoid
Coffee	-	-	-
Artificial sweeteners	-	-	-
Contaminants	Minimize	-	-
Additives	Continue to evaluate	-	-
Vitamin E	-	-	-

Note: a dash (-) indicates that no recommendation has been made.

cancer incidence in the United States by 50% by the year 2000 (113). This prevention awareness endeavor includes a consumer booklet providing dietary recommendations to reduce cancer risk (114). This NCI booklet incorporates and expands on the NAS guidelines and utilizes the format of the original 1981 ACS-funded consumer booklet.

In the wake of the NAS report, and largely in response to it, the American Cancer Society announced its own dietary recommendations in early 1984. These were similar to those of the NAS and NCI. The ACS national headquarters now provides a professional education document on nutrition and cancer (115), and has plans for public education materials in the near future. The California Division of ACS has published a concise public education pamphlet based on the national organization's dietary recommendations (116).

Within five years after Congress raised the question about the relationship between diet and cancer, three prestigious national agencies produced dietary recommendations for the public. Table 1 summarizes and compares these three sets of recommendations which are now a reference point for health professionals and the public. These recommendations have emerged at a relatively rapid pace compared to the usual speed of large bureaucratic organizations. This is especially remarkable given the complex scientific and politically sensitive issue of food and cancer. The combination of research findings, public interest, and the support of key scientists and policy-makers were important factors in this rapid emergence. Another significant factor was that these recommendations were largely consistent with those made for the prevention of heart disease, and the well-known *Dietary Guidelines for Americans* (117). These similarities will help alleviate public confusion and strengthen the nutrition message for preventing chronic diseases and promoting good health.

REFERENCES

1. American Cancer Society, *1984 Cancer Facts and Figures.* American Cancer Society, National Headquarters, New York, 1984.
2. E. Wynder and G. Gori, Contribution of the environment to cancer incidence: An epidemiologic exercise. *J. Natl. Cancer Inst.* **58**, 825–832 (1977).
3. Ibid.
4. R. R. Doll and R. Peto, The causes of cancer: Quantitative estimates of avoidable risks of cancer in the United States today. *J. Natl. Cancer Inst.,* **66**, 1191–1308 (1981).
5. Committee on Diet, Nutrition and Cancer; National Research Council, *Diet, Nutrition, and Cancer.* National Academy Press, Washington, D.C., 1982.

6. G. H. Beaton, J. Milner, V. McGuire, T. E. Feather, and J. A. Little, Source of variance in 24-hour dietary recall data: implications for nutrition study design and interpretation. Carbohydrate sources, vitamins, and minerals. *Am. J. Clin. Nutr.* **37**, 986–995 (1983).

7. J. H. Hankin, A. M. Y. Nomura, J. Lee, T. Hirohata, and L. N. Kolonel, Reproducibility of a diet history questionnaire in a case-control study of breast cancer. *Am. J. Clin. Nutr.* **37**, 981–985 (1983).

8. G. Block, A review of validations of dietary assessment methods. *Am. J. Epidemiol.* **115**, 492–505 (1982).

9. G. H. Beaton, J. Milner, P. Corey et al., Sources of variation in 24-hour dietary recall data: Implications for nutrition study design and interpretation. *Am. J. Clin. Nutr.* **32**, 2546–59 (1979).

10. P. A. Stefanik and M. C. Trulson, Determining the frequency intakes of foods in large group studies. *Am. J. Clin. Nutr.* **11**, 335–43 (1962).

11. B. S. Burke, The dietary history as a tool in research. *J. Am. Diet. Assoc.* **23**, 1041–6 (1947).

12. B. N. Ames, Dietary Carcinogens and Anticarcinogens. *Science* **221**, Sept. 23, 1983, pp. 1256–1264.

13. B. S. Drasar and D. Irving, Environmental factors and cancer of the colon and breast. *Br. J. Cancer* **27**, 167–172 (1973).

14. K. K. Carroll and H. T. Khor, Dietary fat in relation to tumorigenesis. *Prog. Biochem. Pharmacol.* **10**, 308–353 (1975).

15. B. Armstrong and R. Doll, Environmental factors and cancer incidence and mortality in different countries, with special reference to dietary practices. *Int. J. Cancer* **15**, 617–631 (1975).

16. G. Hems, Association between breast cancer mortality rates, child-bearing and diet in the United Kingdom. *Br. J. Cancer* **41**, 429–437 (1980).

17. L. N. Kolonel, J. H. Hankin, J. Lee, S. Y. Chu, A. M. Y. Nomura, and M. W. Hinds, Nutrient intakes in relation to cancer incidence in Hawaii. *Br. J. Cancer* **44**, 332–339 (1981).

18. A. Tannenbaum, The genesis and growth of tumors. III. Effects of a high-fat diet. *Cancer Res.* **2**, 468–475 (1942).

19. K. K. Carroll, Lipids and carcinogenesis. *J. Environ. Pathol. Toxicol.* **3**(4), 253–271 (1980).

20. C. Ip, Ability of dietary fat to overcome the resistance of mature female rats to 7,12-dimethylbenz(a)anthracine-induced mammary tumorigenesis. *Cancer Res.* **40**, 2785–2789 (1980).

21. R. L. Phillips, Role of life-style and dietary habits in risk of cancer among Seventh-Day Adventists. *Cancer Res.* **35**, 3513–3522 (1975).

22. A. B. Miller, A. Kelley, N. W. Choi, V. Matthews, R. W. Morgan, L. Munan, J. D. Burch, J. Feather, G. R. Howe, and M. Jain, A study of diet and breast cancer. *Am. J. Epidemiol.* **107**, 499–509 (1978).

23. C. H. Lingeman, Etiology of cancer of the human ovary: A review. *J. Natl. Cancer Inst.* **53**, 1603–1618 (1974).

24. T. Hirayama, Changing patterns of cancer in Japan with special reference to the decrease in stomach cancer mortality. In H. H. Hiatt, J. D. Watson, and J. A. Winsten, eds., *Origins of Human Cancer, Book A: Incidence of Cancer in Humans.* Cold Spring Harbor Laboratory, Cold Spring Harbor, N.Y., 1977, pp. 55–75.

25. A. J. Lea, Neoplasms and environmental factors. *Annals of the Royal College of Surgery, Engl.* **41**, 432–438 (1967).

26. I. D. Rotkin, Studies in the epidemiology of prostate cancer: Expanded sampling. *Cancer Treatment Rep.* **61**, 173–180 (1977).

27. L. M. Schuman, J. S. Mandell, A. Radke, U. Seal, and F. Halberg, Some selected features of the epidemiology of prostatic cancer: Minneapolis–St. Paul, Minnesota case-control study, 1976–1979. In K. Magnus, ed., *Trends in Cancer Incidence: Causes and Practical Implications* Hemisphere Publishing, Washington, D.C., 1982, pp. 345–354.

28. M. Jain, G. M. Cook, F. G. Davis, M. G. Grace, G. R. How, and A. B. Miller, A case-control study of diet and colorectal cancer. *Int. J. Cancer* **26**, 757–768 (1980).

29. L. G. Dales, G. D. Friedman, H. K. Ury, S. Grossman, and S. R. Williams, A case-control study of relationships of diet and other traits to colorectal cancer in American blacks. *Am. J. Epidemiology* **109**, 132–144 (1978).

30. B. S. Reddy, A. R. Hedges, K. Laakso, and E. L. Wynder, Metabolic epidemiology of large bowel cancer: Fecal bulk and constituents of high-risk North American and low-risk Finnish population. *Cancer* **42**, 2832–2838 (1978).

31. B. S. Reddy, L. A. Cohen, G. D. McCoy, P. Hill, J. H. Weisburger, and E. L. Wynder, Nutrition and its relationship to cancer. *Adv. Cancer Res.* **32**, 237–345 (1980).

32. G. V. Vahouny, M. M. Cassidy, F. Lightfoot, L. Grau, and D. Kritchevsky, Ultrastructural modifications of intestinal and colonic mucosa induced by free or bound bile acids. *Cancer Res.* **41**, 3764–3765 (1981).

33. T. Narisawa, N. E. Magadia, J. H. Weisburger, and E. L. Wynder, Promoting effect of bile acids on colon carcinogenesis after intrarectal instillation of N-methyl-N-nitro-N-nitrosoguanidine in rats. *J. Natl. Cancer Inst.* **53**, 1093–1097 (1974).

34. C. Chomchai, N. Bhadrachari, and N. D. Nigro, The effect of bile on the induction of experimental intestinal tumors in rats. *Dis. Colon Rectum* **17**, 310–312 (1974).

35. R. C. N. Williamson, F. L. R. Bauer, J. S. Ross, J. B. Watkins, and R. A. Malt, Enhanced colonic carcinogenesis with azoxymethane in rats after pancreactico biliary diversion at mid small bowel. *Gastroenterology* **76**, 1388–1392 (1979).

36. C. E. Woteki, M. G. Kovar, and H. Riddick, Sources of differences in estimates of fat intake in national surveys. Paper presented at the 68th Annual Meeting of the Federation of American Societies for

Experimental Biology, St. Louis, Missouri, April 3, 1984.

37. U.S. Congress, Senate, Select Committee on Nutrition and Human Needs. *Dietary Goals for the United States,* 2nd ed., U.S. Government Printing Office, Washington, D.C., December 1977.

38. D. P. Burkitt and H. C. Trowell. *Refined Carbohydrate Foods and Disease. Some Implications of Dietary Fiber.* Academic Press, New York, 1975.

39. K. Liu, J. Stamler, D. Moss, D. Garside, V. Persky, and I. Soltero, Dietary cholesterol, fat, fibre and colon-cancer mortality. *Lancet* 2, 782–785 (1979).

40. O. Manousos, N. E. Day, D. Trichopoulos, F. Gerovassilis, A. Tzonou, and A. Polychronopoulou, Diet and colorectal cancer: a case-control study in Greece. *Int. J. Cancer* 32, 1–5 (1983).

41. B. Modan, V. Barell, F. Lubin, M. Modan, R. A. Greenberg, and S. Grahm, Low-fiber intake as an etiologic factor in cancer of the colon. *J. Natl. Cancer Inst.* 55, 15–18 (1975).

42. L. G. Dales, G. D. Friedman, H. K. Ury, S. Grossman, and S. R. Williams, A case-control study of relationships of diet and other traits to colorectal cancer in American blacks, *Am. J. Epidemiol.* 109, 132–144 (1978).

43. I. Martínez, R. Torres, Z. Frías, J. R. Colón, and M. Fernández, Factors associated with adenocarcinomas of the large bowel in Puerto Rico. In J. M. Birch, ed., *Advances in Medical Oncology, Research and Education. Volume 3: Epidemiology.* Pergamon Press, New York, 1979.

44. D. M. Fleiszer, D. Murray, G. K. Richards, and R. Z. Brown, Effects of diet on chemically induced bowel cancer. *Can. J. Surg.* 23, 67–73 (1980).

45. H. J. Freeman, G. A. Spiller, and Y. S. Kim, A double-blind study on the effects of differing purified cellulose and pectin fiber diets on 1,2-dimethydrazine-induced rat colonic neoplasia. 1980. *Cancer Res.* 40, 2661–2665 (1980).

46. S. Bingham, D. R. R. Williams, T. J. Cole, and W. P. T. James, Dietary fibre and regional large-bowel cancer mortality in Britain. *Br. J. Cancer* 40, 456–463 (1979).

47. G. Kvåle, E. Bjelke, and J. J. Gart, Dietary habits and lung cancer risk. *Int. J. Cancer* 31, 397–405 (1983).

48. E. Bjelke, Dietary vitamin A and human lung cancer. *Int. J. Cancer* 15, 561–565 (1975).

49. C. Mettlin, S. Graham, and M. Swanson, Vitamin A and lung cancer. *J. Natl. Cancer Inst.* 62, 1435–1438 (1979).

50. R. B. Shekelle, S. Liu, W. J. Raynor, Jr., M. Lepper, C. Maliza, and A. H. Rossof, Dietary vitamin A and risk of cancer in the Western Electric Study. *Lancet* 2, 1185–1189 (1981).

51. C. Mettlin and S. Graham, Dietary risk factors in human bladder cancer. *Am. J. Epidemiology* 110, 255–263 (1979).

52. E. Bjelke, Dietary factors and the epidemiology of cancer of the stomach and large bowel. *Aktuel. Ernaehrungsmed. Klin. Prax. Suppl.* 2, 10–17 (1978).

53.   S. Graham, C. Mettlin, J. Marshall, R. Priore, and D. Shedd, Dietary factors in the epidemiology of cancer of the larynx. *Am. J. Epidemiology* **113**, 675–680 (1981).

54.   C. Mettlin, S. Graham, J. Marshall, and M. Swanson, Diet and cancer of the esophagus. *Nutr. Cancer* **2**, 143–147 (1981).

55.   T. Hirayama, Changing patterns of cancer in Japan with special reference to the decrease in stomach cancer mortality. In H. H. Hiatt, J. D. Watson, and J. A. Winsten, eds., *Origins of Human Cancer, Book A: Incidence of Cancer in Humans* Cold Spring Harbor Laboratory, Cold Spring Harbor, N.Y., 1977, pp. 55–75.

56.   P. Nettesheim and M. L. Williams, The influence of vitamin A on the susceptibility of the rat lung to 3-methylcholanthrene. *Int. J. Cancer* **17**, 351–357 (1976).

57.   S. M. Cohen, J. F. Wittenberg, and G. T. Bryan, Effect of avitaminosis A and hypervitaminosis A on urinary bladder carcinogenicity of *N*-[4-(5-nitro-2-furyl)-2-thiazolyl]formamide. *Cancer Res.* **36**, 2334–2339 (1976).

58.   T. Narisawa, B. S. Reddy, C.-Q. Wong, and J. H. Weisberger, Effect of vitamin A deficiency on rat colon carcinogenesis by *N*-methyl-*N*-nitro-*N*-nitrosoguanidine. *Cancer Res.* **36**, 1379–1383 (1976).

59.   R. J. Shamberger, Inhibitory effect of vitamin A on carcinogenesis. *J. Natl. Cancer Inst.* **47**, 667–673 (1971).

60.   A. E. Rogers, B. J. Herndon, and P. M. Newburn, Induction by dimethylhydrazine of intestinal carcinoma in normal rats and rats fed high or low levels of vitamin A. *Cancer Res.* **33**, 1003–1009 (1973).

61.   M. B. Sporn and D. L. Newton, Chemoprevention of cancer with retinoids. *Fed. Proc.* **38**, 2528–2534 (1979).

62.   M. B. Sporn and D. L. Newton, Recent advances in the use of retinoids for cancer prevention. In J. H. Burchenal and F. P. Oettgen, eds., *Cancer. Achievements, Challenges and Prospects for the 1980s*, Vol. 1, Grune and Stratton, New York, 1981, pp. 541–548.

63.   C. H. Hennekens, Physicians Health Study Research Group. Strategies for a primary prevention trial of cancer and cardiovascular disease among U.S. physicians (Abstract). *Am. J. Epidemiol.* **118**, 453–4 (1983).

64.   W. Haenzel and P. Correa, Developments in the epidemiology of stomach cancer over the past decade. *Cancer Res.* **35**, 3452–3459 (1975).

65.   C. Mettlin, S. Graham, R. Priore, J. Marshall, and M. Swanson, Diet and cancer of the esophagus. *Nutr. Cancer* **2**, 143–147 (1981).

66.   L. N. Kolonel, A. M. Y. Nomura, T. Hirohata, J. H. Hankin, and M. W. Hinds, Association of diet and place of birth with stomach cancer incidence in Hawaii Japanese and Caucasians. *Am. J. Clin. Nutr.* **34**, 2478–2485 (1981).

67.   P. J. Cook-Mozaffari, F. Azordegan, N. E. Day, A. Ressicand, C. Sabai, and B. Aramesh, Oesophageal cancer studies in the Caspian littoral of Iran: Results of a case-control study. *Br. J. Cancer* **39**, 293–309 (1979).

68. S. Graham, C. Mettlin, J. Marshall, R. Priore, T. Rzepka, and D. Shedd, Dietary factors in the epidemiology of cancer of the larynx. *Am. J. Epidemiol.* **113**, 675–680 (1981).

69. T. Logue and D. Frommer, The influence of oral vitamin C supplements on experimental colorectal tumor induction (Abstract). *Austr. N. Z. J. Med.* **10**, 588 (1980).

70. B. S. Reddy and N. Hirota, Effect of dietary ascorbic acid on 1,2-dimethylhydrazine-induced colon cancer in rats. *Fed. Proc.* **38**, 714 (1979) Abstract 2565.

71. G. Kallistratos and E. Fasske, Inhibition of benzo(a)pyrene carcinogenesis in rats with vitamin C. *J. Cancer Res. Clin. Oncol.* **97**, 91–96 (1980).

72. S. S. Mirvish, Inhibition of the formation of carcinogenic N-nitroso compounds by ascorbic acid and other compounds. In J. H. Burchenal and H. F. Oettgen, eds., *Cancer: Achievements, Challenges, and Prospects for the 1980s*, Vol. 1, Grune and Stratton, New York, 1981, pp. 557–587.

73. S. Ivankovic, R. Preussman, D. Schmähl, and J. W. Zeller, Prevention by ascorbic acid on *in vivo* formation of N-nitroso compounds. In P. Bogovski and E. A. Walker, eds., *N-Nitroso Compounds in the Environment.* IARC Scientific Publication No. 9., Intl. Agency for Res. on Cancer, Lyon, France, 1975, pp. 101–102.

74. B. Jansson, M. M. Jacobs, and A. C. Griffin, Gastrointestinal cancer: Epidemiology and experimental studies. *Adv. Exp. Med. Biol.* **91**, 305–322 (1978).

75. G. N. Schrauzer, D. A. White, and C. J. Schneider, Cancer mortality correlation studies. III. Statistical associations with dietary selenium intakes. *Bioinorg. Chem.* **7**, 23–34 (1977).

76. G. N. Schrauzer, D. A. White, and C. J. Schneider, Cancer mortality correlation studies. IV. Associations with dietary intakes and blood levels of certain trace elements, notably Se-antagonists. *Bioinorg. Chem.* **7**, 35–56 (1977).

77. R. J. Shamberger, S. A. Tytko, and C. E. Willis, Antioxidants and cancer. Part VI. Selenium and age-adjusted human cancer mortality. *Arch. Environ. Health* **31**, 231–235 (1976).

78. H. A. Schroeder and M. Mitchener, Selenium and tellurium in mice: Effects on growth, survival, and tumors. *Arch. Environ. Health* **24**, 66–71 (1972).

79. J. R. Harr, J. H. Exon, P. D. Whanger, and P. H. Weswig, Effect of dietary selenium on N-2-fluorenyl-acetamide(FAA)-induced cancer in vitamin E supplemented, selenium depleted, rats. *Clin. Toxicol.* **5**, 187–194 (1972).

80. C. Ip and D. K. Sinha, Enhancement of mammary tumorigenesis by dietary selenium deficiency in rats with a high polyunsaturated fat intake. *Cancer Res.* **41**, 31–34 (1981).

81. A. C. Griffin, Role of selenium in the chemoprevention of cancer. *Adv. Cancer Res.* **29**, 419–442 (1979).

82. C. D. Thomson and M. F. Robinson, Selenium in human health and disease with emphasis on those aspects peculiar to New Zealand. *Am. J. Clin. Nutr.* **33**, 303–323 (1980).

83. S. Graham, H. Dayal, M. Swanson, A. Mittelman, and G. Wilkinson, Diet in the epidemiology of cancer of the colon and rectum. *J. Natl. Cancer Inst.* **51**, 709–714 (1978).

84. W. Haenszel, F. B. Locke, and M. Segi, A case-control study of large bowel cancer in Japan. *J. Natl. Cancer Inst.* **64**, 17–22 (1980).

85. W. Lijinsky and A. E. Ross, Production of carcinogenic polynuclear hydrocarbons in the cooking of food. *Food Cosmet. Toxicol.* **5**, 343–347 (1967).

86. C. Lintas, M. C. De Matthaeis, and F. Merli, Determination of benzo(a)pyrene in smoked, cooked and toasted food products. *Food Cosmet. Toxicol.* **17**, 325–328 (1979).

87. T. Sugimura and S. Sato, Mutagens-carcinogens in food. *Cancer Res.* (suppl.) **43**, 2415s (1983).

88. J. W. Howard and T. Fazio, Analytical methodology and reported findings of polycyclic aromatic hydrocarbons in foods. *J. Assoc. Off. Anal. Chem.* **63**, 1077–1104 (1980).

89. L. F. Bjeldanes, M. M. Morris, J. S. Felton, S. Healy, D. Stuermer, P. Berry, H. Timourian, and F. T. Hatch, Mutagens from the cooking of food. II. Survey by Ames/*Salmonella* test of mutagen formation in the major protein-rich foods of the American diet. *Food Chem. Toxicol.* **20**, 357 (1982).

90. B. MacMahon, S. Yen, D. Trichopoulos, K. Warren, and G. Nardi, Coffee and cancer of the pancreas. *N. Engl. J. Med.* **304**, 630–633 (1981).

91. R. S. Lin and I. I. Kessler, A multifactorial model for pancreatic cancer in man: Epidemiological evidence. *J. Am. Med. Assoc.* **245**, 147–152 (1981).

92. H. U. Aeschbacher and W. P. Wurzner, An evaluation of instant and regular coffee in the Ames mutagenicity test. *Toxicol. Lett.* **5**, 139–145 (1980).

93. H.-P. Wurzner, E. Lindstrom, L. Vuataz, and H. Luginbuhl, A two-year feeding study of instant coffee in rats. II. Incidence and types of neoplasms. *Food Cosmet. Toxicol.* **15**, 289–296 (1977).

94. B. C. Challis and C. D. Bartlett, Possible cocarcinogenic effects of coffee constituents. *Nature* **254**, 532–533 (1975).

95. F. Hakulinen, L. Lehtimaki, M. Lehtonen, and L. Teppo, Cancer morbidity among two male cohorts with increased alcohol consumption in Finland. *J. Natl. Cancer Inst.* **52**, 1711–1714 (1974).

96. I. D. J. Bross and J. Coombs, Early onset of oral cancer among women who drink and smoke. *Oncology* **33**, 136–139 (1976).

97. J. D. Burch, G. R. Howe, A. B. Miller, and R. Semenciw, Tobacco, alcohol, asbestos, and nickel in the etiology of cancer of the larynx: a case-control study. *J. Natl. Cancer Inst.* **67**, 1219–1224 (1981).

98. D. Schottenfeld, Alcohol as a cofactor in the etiology of cancer. *Cancer* **43**, 1962–1966 (1979).

99. M. Keller, D. M. Promisel, D. Spiegler, L. Light, and M. N. Davies, eds., Alcohol and cancer. In *Second Special Report to the U.S. Congress on Alcohol and Health.* Public Health Service, DHEW, Rockville, Md., 1977, pp. 53–67.

100. J. Hoey, C. Montvernay, and R. Lambert, Wine and tobacco: Risk factors for gastric cancer in France. *Am. J. Epidemiol.* **113**, 668–674 (1981).

101. J. E. Enstrom, Colorectal cancer and beer drinking. *Br. J. Cancer* **35**, 674–683 (1977).

102. E. S. Pollack, A. M. Y. Nomura, L. K. Heilbrun, G. N. Stemmermann, and S. B. Green, Prospective study of alcohol consumption and cancer. *N. Engl. J. Med.* **310**, 617–21 (1984).

103. L. M. Pottern, L. E. Morris, W. J. Blot, R. G. Zeigler, and J. F. Fraumeni, Jr., Esophageal cancer among Black men in Washington, D.C. I. Alcohol, tobacco, and other risk factors. *J. Natl. Cancer Inst.* **67**, 777–783 (1981).

104. G. D. McCoy, C. B. Chen, S. S. Hecht, and E. C. McCoy, Enhanced metabolism and mutagenesis of nitrosopyrolidine in liver fractions isolated from chronic ethanol-consuming hamsters. *Cancer Res.* **39**, 793–796 (1979).

105. E. A. Lew and L. Garfield, Variations in mortality by weight among 750,000 men and women. *J. Chronic Dis.* **32**, 563–576 (1979).

106. F. de Waard and E. A. Baanders-van Halewijn, A prospective study in general practice on breast-cancer risk in postmenopausal women. *Int. J. Cancer* **14**, 153–160 (1974).

107. F. de Waard, Breast cancer incidence and nutritional status with particular reference to body weight and height. *Cancer Res.* **35**, 3351–6 (1975).

108. G. N. Wogan, Aflatoxin carcinogenesis, In H. Busch, ed., *Methods in Cancer Research, Volume 7.* Academic Press, New York, 1973, pp. 309–344.

109. Committee on Diet, Nutrition, and Cancer; National Research Council, *Diet, Nutrition, and Cancer: Directions for Research.* National Academy Press, Washington, D.C., 1982.

110. W. C. Willett and B. MacMahon, Diet and Cancer—An Overview (Part I). *N. Engl. J. Med.* **310**, 633–38 (1984).

111. W. C. Willett and B. MacMahon, Diet and Cancer—An Overview (Part II). *N. Engl. J. Med.* **310**, 697–703 (1984).

112. C. DiSogra and L. Groll, *Nutrition and Cancer Prevention: A Guide to Food Choices.* Northern California Cancer Program, Palo Alto, Calif., 1981.

113. L. Light, The role of diet in cancer control. Paper presented at the 17th Annual Meeting of the Society for Nutrition Education, Philadelphia, July 11, 1984.

114. National Cancer Institute, *Diet, Nutrition, and Cancer Prevention: A Guide to Food Choices.* Office of Cancer Communications, National Cancer Institute, Bethesda, Md., 1984.

115. American Cancer Society, *Nutrition and Cancer: Cause and Prevention. An American Cancer Society Special Report.* American Cancer Society National Headquarters, New York, 1984.

116. American Cancer Society, *Nutrition and Cancer: Cause and Prevention.* American Cancer Society, California Division, Inc., Oakland, Calif., 1984 (pamphlet).

117. U.S. Dept. of Agriculture and U.S. Dept. of Health, Education, and Welfare, *Nutrition and Your Health, Dietary Guidelines for Americans.* U.S. Government Printing Office, Washington, D.C., February 1980.

2
Dietary Fat and Breast Cancer

KENNETH K. CARROLL, Ph.D.
Department of Biochemistry
University of Western Ontario
London, Ontario, Canada

Address correspondence to Kenneth K. Carroll, Ph.D., Department of Biochemistry, University of Western Ontario, London, Ontario, Canada, N6A 5C1. Kenneth K. Carroll is Professor of Biochemistry and Career Investigator of the Medical Research Council of Canada.

ABSTRACT

Breast cancer causes high mortality among women of many industrialized countries but is less common elsewhere. Mortality is positively correlated with dietary fat, and this correlation is supported by studies on experimental animals. Polyunsaturated fats enhance mammary tumorigenesis in animals more effectively than do saturated fats, but total dietary fat shows the best correlation with breast cancer in humans. Dietary fat appears to act as a promoter of tumor development rather than as a carcinogen. The mechanism for this is not known, but continuous feeding of a high-fat diet appears necessary for maximum effect. Reducing the level of dietary fat two months after treatment of rats with a carcinogen prevented development of many potential tumors. Decreasing fat intake might also reduce breast cancer incidence in human populations and help to prevent recurrence in cancer patients. A reduction in dietary fat might also decrease the incidence of other chronic diseases, including heart disease and certain other types of cancer. The advantages of decreasing dietary fat intake appear to outweigh the disadvantages for most segments of the population. Visible fats and oils, meat, and dairy products account for most of the fat in the American diet. In attempting to reduce fat intake, care should be taken to maintain a balanced diet and to avoid deficiencies of essential nutrients provided by these dietary components.

BACKGROUND

In recent years, breast cancer has caused more deaths in women of the United States and Canada than any other type of cancer (1,2), and the annual mortality shows no sign of decreasing. It is also a major health problem in Australia, New Zealand, and the industrialized countries of Western Europe (3).

In other parts of the world, breast cancer is much less common. For example, until recently, the death rate from breast cancer in Japan was only about one-fifth of that in the United States (3). The lower death

30

rate in Japan is evidently not due to genetic differences, since Japanese immigrants to the United States show a gradual increase in breast cancer mortality, which eventually approaches the rate for other American women (4). Studies on these and other immigrants have led to the concept that environmental factors are largely responsible for observed geographical differences in cancer incidence and mortality (5).

Dietary fat is thought to be one of the more important environmental factors affecting the incidence of breast cancer. This idea is based on epidemiological data from human populations and also on the results of studies on effects of diet on mammary tumors in animals. The evidence has been discussed in a number of earlier reviews (1–3,6–12).

This article provides a summary of some of the earlier work and includes a discussion of the effects of different types of dietary fat. Evidence that dietary fat acts mainly at the promotional stage of mammary carcinogenesis is also described. This concept has important implications since it suggests the possibility that reducing dietary fat intake, besides decreasing the risk of developing breast cancer, might also help to delay or prevent recurrence of the disease in breast cancer patients.

Consideration of the sources of fat in the American diet gives an indication of dietary changes that would be required to achieve a substantial reduction in dietary fat intake. Possible benefits and disadvantages associated with such a reduction are also discussed.

EVIDENCE RELATING DIETARY FAT TO BREAST CANCER

Epidemiological data show a strong positive correlation between mortality from breast cancer in different countries and the amount of fat per capita available for consumption in those countries (Fig. 1). This does not necessarily mean that breast cancer develops more readily because of high fat consumption, but studies on rats and mice have consistently shown that animals fed high-fat diets develop mammary tumors more readily than those fed low-fat diets. This applies to both spontaneous tumors and tumors induced by various chemical carcinogens or by irradiation (12). Thus, the results of experiments with animals support the positive correlation observed in epidemiologic data on human populations.

Case-control studies have shown only a weak association between breast cancer and consumption of high-fat foods (13,14), but this may be because dietary variations among individuals living in the same or nearby communities are smaller than those among people living in

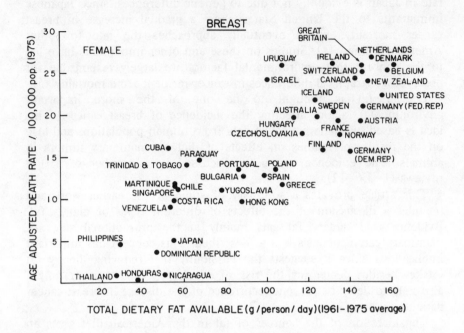

Fig 1. Correlation between age-adjusted mortality from breast cancer and the total dietary fat available for consumption in different countries (from reference 12).

different countries. It is also difficult in such studies to obtain accurate information on past dietary histories that may be relevant to development of breast cancer.

Fat is a more concentrated source of calories than either carbohydrate or protein, and the caloric intake in different countries shows a positive correlation with breast cancer mortality similar to that observed for dietary fat. The same can be said for animal protein, which tends to be closely correlated with dietary fat in human diets (6).

It is difficult to dissociate these dietary variables in studies on human populations. However, experiments with animals have provided evidence that dietary fat exerts an effect on mammary tumorigenesis independent of caloric intake, and there is little evidence from animal experiments to indicate that mammary carcinogenesis is correlated with intake of animal protein (7).

EFFECTS OF DIFFERENT TYPES OF DIETARY FAT

Our first experiment dealing with effects of dietary fat on mammary tumorigenesis induced in female Sprague–Dawley rats by 7,12-dimethylbenz(α)anthracene (DMBA) showed that rats fed a semipurified diet containing 20%, by weight, corn oil developed twice as many tumors as rats fed similar diets containing either 0.5% corn oil or 20% coconut oil (15). Further experiments in which a variety of different fats and oils were fed at the 20% level provided additional evidence that unsaturated oils markedly increased the tumor yield, whereas saturated fats had little or no effect (6,16). Since the unsaturated oils were mostly of plant origin and contained no cholesterol, this indicated that the effect was not due to dietary cholesterol. A recent report by Cohen and Chan (17) likewise showed that dietary cholesterol has little effect on mammary tumorigenesis in rats.

The differing effects of saturated and unsaturated fats in our experiments appear to be related to differences in their content of polyunsaturated essential fatty acids. When coconut oil or beef tallow (largely saturated) was supplemented with corn oil or sunflower-seed oil (largely polyunsaturated), feeding the mixtures as 20% by weight of the diet increased the yield of tumors as effectively as feeding the polyunsaturated oils themselves at the same level (12,16,18). The essential fatty acid, linoleic acid (polyunsaturated), fed as the ethyl ester, was as effective as the corn oil or sunflower-seed oil, whereas adding the same amount of ethyl oleate (monounsaturated) to a high coconut oil diet produced no increase in tumor yield (16).

These experiments indicated a requirement for polyunsaturated fatty acids as well as a high-fat diet for enhancement of tumorigenesis in the DMBA-tumor model. At intermediate levels of dietary fat (10% by weight), polyunsaturated fats such as corn oil and sunflower-seed oil still produced a marked enhancement of tumor yield, but when lesser amounts of these fats (3% by weight) were added to saturated fats and the mixtures fed as 10% by weight, they failed to increase the tumor yield above that observed with the low-fat diet (12,18).

The effects of other constituents of dietary fats, such as tocopherols, have not been investigated specifically in our experiments. Ip (19) reported that vitamin E deficiency increased the yield of mammary tumors, but feeding amounts in excess of normal requirements did not inhibit tumorigenesis. Variable effects have been observed with other antioxidants (20).

In view of the results obtained in experiments with animals, it is of interest to know how well breast cancer mortality in humans correlates with different types of dietary fat. When mortality was plotted against dietary fat available from either animal or plant sources, it was observed that the correlation with animal fat was about as strong as that for total fat, whereas dietary vegetable oils showed no correlation with breast cancer mortality (7,16). In general, vegetable oils tend to be more unsaturated than animal fats and, although they are often hydrogenated for use in food products, these epidemiological data did not at first seem to be in agreement with the results of our experiments with animals.

It seems possible, however, that the requirement for polyunsaturated fatty acids may be satisfied by most national diets, and the observed positive correlation between dietary fat and breast cancer mortality may therefore be related mainly to the other significant variable in the animal experiments, which is the total amount of fat in the diet. Thus, the epidemiological data are not necessarily at variance with results obtained with the animal model.

It must also be kept in mind that the epidemiological data are relatively crude with respect to both the mortality figures and the amounts of fat available for consumption. Thus, although such data serve a useful purpose in pointing the way to possible meaningful relationships, the evidence must be interpreted with caution. It is largely the supporting data from animal experiments that lend significance to the observed correlation between dietary fat and breast cancer in human populations.

DIETARY FAT AS A PROMOTER OF MAMMARY TUMORIGENESIS

In our initial studies on the effects of dietary fat on mammary tumorigenesis in rats, the animals were fed semipurified diets containing various types and levels of dietary fat from the time of weaning and were given a single dose of DMBA at 50 days of age. They were then continued on the respective diets, and the development of tumors was followed over a period of about four months. One of the advantages of animal models for mammary cancer is that the tumors can be palpated as small, hard lumps at a very early stage in their development, so the process of tumorigenesis can be followed without killing the animals.

In an early attempt to obtain information on the mechanism by which dietary fat affects mammary carcinogenesis, a crossover experiment was carried out in which rats were switched from a low-fat diet to a high-fat diet or vice versa at the time of treatment with DMBA. Control groups were fed the high-fat diet or the low-fat diet both before and after receiving the DMBA. The results of this experiment showed a higher incidence of tumors in rats fed the high-fat diet after DMBA, regardless of the level of fat fed before the carcinogen was given (6).

In a subsequent experiment, all of the rats were fed a low-fat, semipurified diet until after treatment with DMBA. One group was then continued on the low-fat diet as a control, while other groups were switched to a high-fat diet 1, 2, or 4 weeks later. This experiment showed that the tumor yield was markedly increased in the groups switched to a high-fat diet 1 or 2 weeks after exposure to DMBA, but rats changed to a high-fat diet after 4 weeks developed only as many tumors as those that continued on the low-fat diet throughout (6).

The above results suggested that dietary fat was acting as a promoting agent rather than affecting initiation of tumors, although it seemed to be most effective during the early period after treatment with the carcinogen. The fact that dietary fat has been observed to increase the yield of spontaneous tumors as well as tumors induced by various chemical or physical agents is a further indication that it is acting as a promoting agent rather than affecting the process of initiation (12,18).

Experiments in other laboratories have provided additional support for this conclusion. Hopkins and West (21) studied the effects of dietary fat on a transplantable mammary tumor in mice. They prepared a suspension of dissociated tumor cells and, by injecting varying quantities of cells, determined the number that would produce tumors in half of the mice injected. They then gave this number of tumor cells to mice fed either a high-saturated or a high-polyunsaturated fat diet, and found that a larger proportion of mice fed the high-polyunsaturated fat diet developed tumors. Similar studies in our laboratory with the same transplantable tumor showed that mice fed a high-fat diet developed tumors more readily than those fed a low-fat diet (G. J. Hopkins and K. K. Carroll, unpublished experiments).

The studies of Abraham and his colleagues on transplantable tumors in mice and rats also support the concept that dietary fat acts as a promoter of mammary tumorigenesis (22,23). In their experiments, however, comparisons were usually made between diets devoid of essential fatty acids and diets containing varying amounts of added essential fatty acids or polyunsaturated fats. This is somewhat different from our studies in which the low fat diets or diets containing relatively saturated fats might contain appreciable amounts of essential fatty acids without producing any apparent enhancement of tumor yield, whereas diets containing larger amounts of essential fatty acids or higher levels of dietary fat substantially increased the number of tumors that developed.

POSSIBLE MECHANISMS INVOLVED IN PROMOTION OF MAMMARY CARCINOGENESIS BY DIETARY FAT

It seems probable from the above experiments that dietary fat exerts its main effect at the promotional stage of mammary carcinogenesis, but there are still many ways in which this effect could be mediated. Some of the possibilities include: changes in the hormonal environment, alterations in the fatty acid composition of cellular membranes, modification of immune responses, effects mediated by physiologically active oxidation products of fatty acids, and alterations in cellular metabolic pathways.

Chan and Cohen proposed on the basis of their studies that dietary fat influenced mammary tumorigenesis by increasing the ratio of prolactin to estrogen in the circulation during the proestrus—estrus phase of the cycle (24). Subsequent studies have provided evidence both for and against this hypothesis (16,18). In their experiments, Chan and Cohen measured the circulating hormone levels in blood drawn from rats under ether anesthesia, which is known to produce a marked stimulation of prolactin secretion. In our studies, which failed to show a positive correlation between the prolactin—estrogen ratio and mammary tumorigenesis, the blood was collected following decapitation of the rats in order to avoid any stimulatory effect on prolactin secretion (3). Possibly the relationship only applies under conditions in which prolactin secretion is strongly stimulated. There is some evidence that diet can affect nocturnal release of prolactin in human subjects (25).

The role of prolactin in tumorigenesis is not well understood. Under some conditions it appears to act as a promoter, but in other situations it can inhibit mammary tumorigenesis (26). Estrogens can produce mammary tumors in animals (27), but there is still much uncertainty about their relationship to breast cancer in humans (28).

Normal development of the mammary gland is undoubtedly influenced by hormones, and mammary tumors are often hormone dependent. Dietary fat may influence mammary carcinogenesis through a hormonal mechanism, but the relationship could be more subtle than a simple correlation with circulating levels of hormones. There is evidence that mammary tumors contain higher levels of estrogen and prolactin receptors in rats fed high-fat diets compared to those fed very low-fat diets, but it is still not clear whether this can account for the observed differences in susceptibility to tumorigenesis (29).

As discussed earlier, our studies have indicated that enhancement of mammary tumorigenesis by dietary fat is dependent on both the type and amount of dietary fat. It appears that part of the effect is related to a requirement for essential fatty acids. Normal development of the mammary gland is dependent on an adequate supply of essential fatty acids (30), and it is to be expected that abnormal growth would be influenced in a similar way. Essential fatty acids are components of the membrane phospholipids of all cells and are thus required for cellular proliferation. Whether this requirement is sufficient to explain the enhancement of mammary tumorigenesis is questionable. Preliminary experiments in our laboratory provided evidence of a positive correlation between the degree of polyunsaturation of mammary tissue phospholipids and the mammary tumor yield in rats fed different types and amounts of fat (3), but this relationship was not consistently observed in subsequent studies (M. B. Davidson and K. K. Carroll, unpublished experiments).

Besides acting as building blocks for cellular membranes, essential fatty acids may influence mammary tumorigenesis in other ways. For example, diets high in polyunsaturated fat have been reported to inhibit cell-mediated immune responses (31), and this could enhance tumor yields by limiting the effectiveness of immune surveillance. Essential fatty acids are also precursors of a wide range of physiologically active products that might influence the process of carcinogenesis. These include prostaglandins, prostacyclin, thromboxanes, leucotrienes, and various hydroperoxides. There is some evidence that prostaglandins can act as promoters (3), and the studies of Abraham and his coworkers with prostaglandin-synthesis inhibitors have provided evidence that prostaglandins are involved in observed effects of dietary fat on growth of their transplantable mammary tumors (22,23). This possibility is obviously worthy of further investigation.

It is less easy to think of ways in which a high-fat diet per se could influence mammary tumorigenesis. This requirement appears to be related in some way to the need for essential fatty acids, since at lower levels of dietary fat a higher degree of polyunsaturation was necessary to enhance the tumor yield (12,18). It seems possible that the effect of dietary fat on mammary tumorigenesis is basically dependent on essential fatty acids or their metabolic products, and that the availability of these substances is affected by the overall amount of fat in the diet.

The level of fat in the diet can, however, markedly influence cellular metabolic patterns, and this could significantly affect growth and proliferation of tumor cells. The rate of flux in pathways such as glycolysis, gluconeogenesis, fatty acid oxidation, and fatty acid biosynthesis is influenced by the relative proportions of fat and carbohydrate in the diet. It is at least conceivable that alterations in these pathways and associated effects on hormones and co-factors due to a high-fat diet might be conducive to tumor development.

REVERSAL OF TUMOR PROMOTION BY REDUCING DIETARY FAT INTAKE

Since dietary fat appears to be acting primarily at the promotional stage of tumorigenesis, it is presumably serving as a stimulant to the growth and proliferation of neoplastic cells rather than affecting their formation. One of the characteristic features of tumor promotion is the need for continued exposure to the promoting agent over prolonged periods of time. It is therefore of interest that the promotional effect of dietary fat can be largely prevented by reducing the fat content of the diet after a period of exposure to a high-fat diet (32–34).

Studies in our laboratory have shown that removal of fat from the diet after seven weeks of promotion by a high-fat diet has a marked inhibitory effect on subsequent growth and development of mammary tumors induced by DMBA (32). Similar observations were made by Ip and Ip (33), who reduced the dietary fat to 0.5% after periods of up to 6 weeks on a high-fat diet. Cohen et al. (35) also observed a marked reduction in mammary tumorigenesis in rats maintained on a low-fat diet compared to those fed a high-fat diet following ovariectomy 80 days after treatment with DMBA.

A more recent experiment in our laboratory has indicated that it is not necessary to reduce the dietary fat to extremely low levels in order to counteract the promotional effect of a high-fat diet on mammary tumorigenesis (34). Rats were treated with DMBA at 50 days of age and, beginning one week later, were fed a diet containing 20% sunflower-seed oil for seven weeks, by which time about one-third of the animals had developed tumors. They were then divided into five groups of 31 rats each, with the tumor-bearers equally distributed among the groups. One group was continued on the 20% sunflower-seed oil diet; one group was given a fat-free diet; and the other three groups were fed diets containing 10% coconut oil, 10% butter, and 10% lard, respectively. Over the next 30 weeks, the group that continued on the sunflower-seed oil diet developed substantially more new tumors than any of the other groups. In fact, the rats fed the butter and lard diets developed only about as many tumors as those on the fat-free diet, while rats on the coconut oil diet had the least number of new tumors (34).

Toward the end of this experiment, some of the rats on the fat-free diet had an elevated triene−tetraene ratio in their plasma fatty acids, indicative of essential fatty acid deficiency. There was, however, no evidence of such a deficiency in any of the other groups. Indeed, the lard used in our experiment contained about 13% linoleic acid, so the inhibition of tumorigenesis could hardly be attributed to a deficiency of essential fatty acids in the usual sense of the term (R. Kalamegham and K. K. Carroll, unpublished data).

GENETIC VERSUS ENVIRONMENTAL FACTORS IN THE DEVELOPMENT OF BREAST CANCER IN HUMANS

Genetic factors no doubt play a role in the development of breast cancer, as indicated by data showing that women having close relatives with breast cancer are at increased risk of developing the disease (36,37). Studies on migrating populations have made it clear, however, that genetic factors alone cannot explain the large geographical differences in breast cancer incidence and mortality. The best-documented studies are those on Japanese immigrants to the United States, who show a marked increase in incidence and mortality from breast cancer over a period of time (4). Similar observations have been made in other migrating populations (5). These changes are presumably due to alterations in lifestyle, of which diet may be the most important.

Within the population of any given country there appear to be a number of factors that influence susceptibility to breast cancer. For example, it has long been recognized that pregnancy exerts a protective effect, and that risk is inversely correlated with age at first birth (37). Such factors may help to determine individual susceptibility to breast cancer, but it seems probable that by altering environmental conditions it should be possible to decrease breast cancer incidence and mortality in American women to rates comparable to those in countries such as Japan. Since mortality from breast cancer in American women is about five times higher than in Japanese women, this represents a potential saving of many lives and much suffering.

REDUCTION OF DIETARY FAT FOR PREVENTION AND TREATMENT OF BREAST CANCER

Evidence accumulating from epidemiological data and from experiments with animals has suggested that differences in dietary fat intake are largely responsible for observed geographical differences in the occurrence of breast cancer. If this is so, a reduction in dietary fat intake should eventually lead to a decrease in breast cancer incidence and mortality. On the basis of such considerations, a substantial reduction in dietary fat intake was recommended by the Committee on Diet, Nutrition, and Cancer in their report to the National Research Council (11).

The rationale for such a recommendation would be greatly enhanced if it could be demonstrated directly in a human population that a reduction in dietary fat is actually followed by a decrease in breast cancer. As indicated above, the reverse has been observed in a number of migrating populations, and it also seems to be happening in present-day Japan, where fat intake is increasing and breast cancer is becoming more prevalent (9). Without better evidence, it may be difficult to persuade a free-living population to reduce their fat intake sufficiently for a long enough period of time to demonstrate a convincing reduction in breast cancer incidence. It might be possible, however, to carry out such an experiment in a population at higher than normal risk, such as women with certain types of benign breast disease (37,38), or women having a number of close relatives with breast cancer (36,37).

Another possibility is suggested by our recent studies on mammary cancer in rats, as described in an earlier section. These studies indicated that reducing the dietary fat from 20 to 10% by weight of the diet (i.e., from approximately 40 to 20% of calories) markedly inhibited development of tumors from initiated cells, even though the fat intake was not reduced until some time after exposure to carcinogen. In women with breast cancer, the main problem is not so much the primary tumor, which can be removed by surgery, but the metastatic lesions which subsequently develop in other parts of the body and which are much more difficult to treat by surgery or other means. If micrometastases behave similarly to the initiated sites in our animal model, it seems possible that their development might be delayed or prevented by reducing the fat intake of the cancer patient as soon as possible after the primary tumor is detected. This need not preclude other forms of treatment.

Because recurrence is rather frequent in women with breast cancer, even when it is detected in the early stages, it might be possible to conduct a meaningful clinical trial with sufficient women in this high-risk group, using recurrence over a five-year period as a means of assessment (39). Since they are at increased risk, it should be relatively easy to obtain compliance with a low-fat diet in such a group. If a low-fat diet could be shown to have a protective effect in a high-risk population, this would provide a much better rationale for recommending a reduction in dietary fat for the population as a whole. In considering the possibility of a dietary trial with breast cancer patients, it is noteworthy that such patients have been observed to have better survival rates in Japan, where breast cancer occurs less frequently (39).

DIETARY FAT IN RELATION TO OTHER TYPES OF CANCER

Epidemiological data have shown strong positive correlations between dietary fat and certain other types of cancer as well, and in some cases the data are supported by results of experiments on animals. Some of the types that show this correlation are often, like breast cancer, responsible for a large proportion of cancer deaths in the more industrialized countries.

Colon cancer in both men and women is positively correlated with dietary fat intake, and there is evidence that rats treated with carcinogens to induce intestinal tumors develop more tumors on a high-fat compared to a low-fat diet (9). Cancer of the prostate, which has a high mortality rate in North American men, also shows a strong positive correlation with dietary fat intake, but in this case the evidence from animal experiments is much more limited (40). Pancreatic cancer is likewise positively correlated with dietary fat intake, and it has recently been shown that rats fed a high-polyunsaturated fat diet develop this type of cancer more readily than those fed a high-saturated fat diet (41).

Cancers at other body sites show varying degrees of correlation with dietary fat, ranging from relatively strong positive correlations for leukemia, aleukemia, and cancers of the rectum and ovary; to no correlation with stomach cancer; and to a negative correlation with liver cancer (6).

POSSIBLE ADVANTAGES AND DISADVANTAGES OF REDUCING DIETARY FAT INTAKE

In making recommendations for dietary changes in populations as a whole, it is important to consider not only the possible benefits that might accrue relative to some particular disease, but also how the changes may affect other diseases and the general health and well-being of the population. A reduction in dietary fat has also been recommended as a means of reducing the risk of cardiovascular disease (42). Furthermore, high-fat diets may contribute to other health problems such as gallstones and diverticular disease (43). Since fat contains more than twice as many calories per gram as either protein or carbohydrate, high-fat diets tend to have high caloric density, and ingestion of such diets may thus contribute to obesity, which is recognized as a major health problem in North America. Thus, a reduction in dietary fat may have benefits other than those relating to cancer incidence and mortality.

Are there also disadvantages in reducing the fat content of the diet? Fat serves mainly as a concentrated source of calories, but in addition it provides fat-soluble vitamins and essential fatty acids, and facilitates the absorption of fat-soluble vitamins from the gut. Symptoms of deficiency of fat-soluble vitamins are not commonly seen in North American populations, but it would be desirable to ensure that the diet is adequately supplemented with these vitamins if dietary fat were substantially reduced.

Symptoms of essential fatty acid deficiency have only rarely been seen in humans (44), and it seems unlikely that a deficiency would occur as a result of reducing dietary fat. In recent years, an increased intake of polyunsaturated fat has been recommended as a means of reducing serum cholesterol levels and protecting against cardiovascular disease (45). There may, however, be contraindications to a high intake of polyunsaturated fat. There is some evidence that it promotes formation of gallstones (46), and experiments in animals have indicated that polyunsaturated fats promote mammary tumorigenesis more effectively than do saturated fats (6). A general reduction in dietary fat is probably preferable to altering the proportions of the different types of fat.

A diet with lower fat content may, however, be less desirable for certain segments of the population. For example, infants under one year of age should probably have a relatively high-fat diet because their high caloric requirement for growth can be more readily met by such a diet. People who are doing heavy physical work or who are habitually exposed to a cold environment may likewise be better off with a diet that is relatively high in fat. For sedentary, middle-aged individuals, however, some reduction in dietary fat would probably be beneficial, since it might decrease susceptibility to a number of chronic diseases, including cancer.

SOURCES OF FAT IN THE AMERICAN DIET

In order to reduce the fat content of the diet it is necessary first to identify the kinds of food that contribute most of the dietary fat. It can be seen from Table 1 that the visible fats and oils used as spreads, cooking fats, and salad oils are the major source of fat, contributing about 40% of the total.

Meats and milk products are the other main sources and, compared to these, most other components contribute relatively little fat. Foods such as eggs and nuts are quite high in fat, but are not normally eaten in sufficient quantities to contribute significantly to dietary fat intake.

Table 1. Sources of Dietary Fat in the United States[a]

Food Group		Fat Calories (Percent of Total)
Cereals		1.5
Roots and tubers		0.1
Nuts and oilseeds		3.6
Vegetables		0.4
Fruits		0.5
Meat		38.0
Cattle	16.8	
Pigs	17.4	
Chickens	2.4	
Egg		2.7
Fish and seafood		0.4
Milk products		12.1
Milk	8.0	
Cheese	3.7	
Oils and fats		39.7
Vegetable		
Margarines, shortenings	16.0	
Soybeans/oil	10.8	
Other	6.2	
Animal		
Butter	2.7	
Lard	2.0	
Other	2.0	
Total dietary fat available		163.9 g/person/day

[a] Average for 1975–77 based on data from FAO (47).

In principle, it should therefore be relatively easy to achieve a substantial reduction in dietary fat intake, but this may be considerably more difficult in practice. Many of our most common foods, including most of the convenience foods and those served at fast food outlets, have a high fat content, and in most restaurants it is difficult to obtain a low-fat meal. Many people therefore consider that it would be difficult to reduce fat consumption even to 30% of total calories. Furthermore, dietary fat improves the texture and palatability of food and provides a sense of satiety that enhances the enjoyment of eating. Increasing affluence is frequently associated with a rise in the fat content of the diet, and any attempt to reverse this trend represents a challenge to nutritionists and food producers.

CONCLUDING REMARKS

Breast cancer continues to be a major cause of death in North American women, and the death rate shows no sign of decreasing in spite of improvements in diagnosis and treatment. Epidemiological data indicate, however, that the death rate from breast cancer is much higher in North America than in many other parts of the world. This difference appears to be related to environment rather than heredity, and there is accumulating evidence that geographical differences in breast cancer mortality are closely related to consumption of dietary fat.

It is evident that some new approaches are required to reduce the death toll from breast cancer. One way might be to reduce the intake of dietary fat. The difficulties of such an approach should not be minimized, but attempts could be made to develop and promote low-fat food products that can compete successfully with the high-fat items that presently make up much of our food supply. Meanwhile, studies on animal models should be continued to define more precisely the effects of dietary fat on mammary tumorigenesis, and to determine the mechanisms involved. Knowledge of these mechanisms might suggest alternative ways of neutralizing the promotional effects of dietary fat on mammary cancer.

ACKNOWLEDGMENTS

Support by the National Cancer Institute of Canada and the contributions of coworkers in our studies on dietary fat in relation to mammary cancer are gratefully acknowledged.

REFERENCES

1. E. L. Wynder, G. D. McCoy, B. S. Reddy, L. Cohen, P. Hill, N. E. Spingarn, and J. H. Weisburger, Nutrition and metabolic epidemiology of cancers of the oral cavity, esophagus, colon, breast, prostate, and stomach. In G. R. Newell and N. M. Ellison, eds., *Progress in Cancer Research and Therapy, Vol. 17. Nutrition and Cancer: Etiology and Treatment,* Raven Press, New York, 1981, p. 11.
2. K. K. Carroll, Dietary fat and its relationship to human cancer. In H. F. Stich, ed., *Carcinogens and Mutagens in the Environment, Vol. I. Food Products,* CRC Press, Inc., Boca Raton, Fla., 1982, p. 31.
3. K. K. Carroll, Neutral fats and cancer. *Cancer Res.* **41**, 3695 (1981).

4.   J. W. Berg, Can nutrition explain the pattern of international epidemiology of hormone-dependent cancers? *Cancer Res.* **35**, 3345 (1975).

5.   G. B. Gori, Diet and nutrition in cancer causation, *Nutr. Cancer* **1**, 5 (1978).

6.   K. K. Carroll and H. T. Khor, Dietary fat in relation to tumorigenesis. *Prog. Biochem. Pharmacol.* **10**, 308 (1975).

7.   K. K. Carroll, Experimental evidence of dietary factors and hormone-dependent cancers. *Cancer Res.* **35**, 3374 (1975).

8.   J. H. Hankin and V. Rawlings, Diet and breast cancer: a review. *Am. J. Clin. Nutr.* **31**, 2005 (1978).

9.   B. S. Reddy, L. A. Cohen, G. D. McCoy, P. Hill, J. H. Weisburger, and E. L. Wynder, Nutrition and its relationship to cancer. *Adv. Cancer Res.* **32**, 237 (1980).

10. K. K. Carroll, Influence of diet on mammary cancer. *Nutr. Cancer* **2**, 232 (1981).

11. Committee on Diet, Nutrition, and Cancer, Assembly of Life Sciences, National Research Council, *Diet, Nutrition, and Cancer,* National Academy Press, Washington, D.C., 1982.

12. K. K. Carroll, The role of dietary fat in carcinogenesis. In E. G. Perkins and W. J. Visek, eds., *AOCS Monograph 10, Dietary Fats and Health,* American Oil Chemists' Society, Champaign, Ill., 1983, p. 710.

13. A. B. Miller, A. Kelly, N. W. Choi, V. Matthews, R. W. Morgan, L. Munan, J. D. Burch, J. Feather, G. R. Howe, and M. Jain, A study of diet and breast cancer. *Am. J. Epidemiol.* **107**, 499 (1978).

14. L. N. Kolonel, A. M. Y. Nomura, M. W. Hinds, T. Hirohata, J. H. Hankin, and J. Lee, Role of diet in cancer incidence in Hawaii. *Cancer Res. Suppl.* **43**, 2397s (1983).

15. E. B. Gammal, K. K. Carroll, and E. R. Plunkett, Effects of dietary fat on mammary carcinogenesis by 7,12-dimethylbenz(α)anthracene in rats, *Cancer Res.* **27**, 1737 (1967).

16. K. K. Carroll, G. J. Hopkins, T. G. Kennedy, and M. B. Davidson, Essential fatty acids in relation to mammary carcinogenesis. *Prog. Lipid Res.* **20**, 685 (1981).

17. L. A. Cohen and P.-C. Chan, Dietary cholesterol and experimental mammary cancer development. *Nutr. Cancer* **4**, 99 (1982).

18. K. K. Carroll and M. B. Davidson, The role of lipids in tumorigenesis. In M. S. Arnott, J. van Eys, and Y.-M. Wang, eds., *Molecular Interrelations of Nutrition and Cancer,* Raven Press, New York, 1982, p. 237.

19. C. Ip, Dietary vitamin E intake and mammary carcinogenesis in rats. *Carcinogenesis* **3**, 1453 (1982).

20. M. M. King and P. B. McCay, Modulation of tumor incidence and possible mechanisms of inhibition of mammary carcinogenesis by dietary antioxidants. *Cancer Res. Suppl.* **43**, 2485s (1983).

21. G. J. Hopkins and C. E. West, Effect of dietary polyunsaturated fat on the

growth of a transplantable adenocarcinoma in C3H^{vy}fB mice. *J. Natl. Cancer Inst.* **58**, 753 (1977).

22. L. A. Hillyard and S. Abraham, Effect of dietary polyunsaturated fatty acids on growth of mammary adenocarcinomas in mice and rats. *Cancer Res.* **39**, 4430 (1979).

23. S. Abraham. In E. G. Perkins, and W. J. Visek, eds., *AOCS Monograph 10, Dietary Fats and Health*, American Oil Chemists' Society, Champaign, Ill., 1983, p. 817.

24. P.-C. Chan and L. A. Cohen, Dietary fat and growth promotion of rat mammary tumors. *Cancer Res.* **35**, 3384 (1975).

25. P. Hill and E. Wynder, Diet and prolactin release. *Lancet* **2**, 806 (1976).

26. C. W. Welsch and H. Nagasawa, Prolactin and murine mammary tumorigenesis: A review. *Cancer Res.* **37**, 951 (1977).

27. R. L. Noble, B. C. Hochachka, and D. King, Spontaneous and estrogen-produced tumors in Nb rats and their behavior after transplantation. *Cancer Res.* **35**, 766 (1975).

28. T. L. Dao, The role of ovarian steroid hormones in mammary carcinogenesis. In M. C. Pike, P. K. Siiteri, and C. W. Welsch, eds., *Banbury Report 8. Hormones and Breast Cancer*, Cold Spring Harbor Laboratory, Cold Spring Harbor, N.Y., 1981, p. 281.

29. C. W. Welsch and C. F. Aylsworth, Enhancement of murine mammary tumorigenesis by feeding high levels of dietary fat: A hormonal mechanism? *JNCI* **70**, 215 (1983).

30. R. A. Knazek and S. C. Liu, Effects of dietary essential fatty acids on murine mammary gland development. *Cancer Res.* **41**, 3750 (1981).

31. J. J. Vitale and S. A. Broitman, Lipids and immune function. *Cancer Res.* **41**, 3706 (1981).

32. M. B. Davidson and K. K. Carroll, Inhibitory effect of a fat-free diet on mammary carcinogenesis in rats. *Nutr. Cancer* **3**, 207 (1982).

33. C. Ip and M. M. Ip, Inhibition of mammary tumorigenesis by a reduction of fat intake after carcinogen treatment in young versus adult rats. *Cancer Lett.* **11**, 35 (1980).

34. K. K. Carroll and R. Kalamegham, Lipid components and cancer. In E. L. Wynder, G. A. Leveille, J. H. Weisburger, and G. E. Livingston, eds., *Environmental Aspects of Cancer: The Role of Macro and Micro Components of Foods*, Food and Nutrition Press, Inc., Westport, Conn., p. 101 (in press).

35. L. A. Cohen, P. C. Chan, and E. L. Wynder, The role of a high-fat diet in enhancing the development of mammary tumors in ovariectomized rats. *Cancer* **47**, 66 (1981).

36. C. D. Haagensen, C. Bodian, and D. E. Haagensen, Jr., *Breast Carcinoma: Risk and Detection*. W. B. Saunders, Philadelphia, 1981, p. 14.

37. B. MacMahon, P. Cole, and J. Brown, Etiology of human breast cancer: A review. *J. Natl. Cancer Inst.* **50**, 21 (1973).

38. N. T. Fleming, B. K. Armstrong, and H. J. Sheiner, The comparative

epidemiology of benign breast lumps and breast cancer in Western Australia. *Int. J. Cancer* **30**, 147 (1982).

39. E. L. Wynder and L. A. Cohen, A rationale for dietary intervention in the treatment of postmenopausal breast cancer patients. *Nutr. Cancer* **3**, 195 (1982).

40. S. Katayama, E. Fiala, B. S. Reddy, A. Rivenson, J. Silverman, G. M. Williams, and J. H. Weisburger, Prostate adenocarcinoma in rats: Induction by 3,2'-dimethyl-4-aminobiphenyl. *JNCI* **68**, 867 (1982).

41. B. D. Roebuck, J. D. Yager, Jr., and D. S. Longnecker, Dietary modulation of azaserine-induced pancreatic carcinogenesis in the rat. *Cancer Res.* **41**, 888 (1981).

42. S. Palmer, Diet, nutrition and cancer: The future of dietary policy. *Cancer. Res. Suppl.* **43**, 2509s (1983).

43. D. P. Burkitt, Western diseases and their emergence related to diet. *S. Afr. Med. J.* **61**, 1013 (1982).

44. R. T. Holman, Essential fatty acid deficiency in humans. In M. Rechcigl, Jr., ed., *Handbook Series in Nutrition and Food. Section E. Nutritional Disorders, Vol. III*, CRC Press, West Palm Beach, Fla., 1978, p. 335.

45. Rationale of the diet-heart statement of the American Heart Association. Report of AHA Nutrition Committee. *Arteriosclerosis* **2**, 177 (1982).

46. R. A. L. Sturdevant, M. L. Pearce, and S. Dayton, Increased prevalence of cholelithiasis in men ingesting a serum-cholesterol-lowering diet. *New Engl. J. Med.* **288**, 24 (1973).

47. *Food Balance Sheets, 1975-77 Average, and Per Caput Food Supplies. 1961-65. Average, 1967 to 1977.* Food and Agriculture Organization of the United Nations, Rome, 1980, p. 941.

48. R. Doll and R. Peto, The causes of cancer: quantitative estimates of avoidable risks of cancer in the United States today. *JNCI* **66**, 1191 (1981).

3
Nutrition and Diabetes

JAMES W. ANDERSON, M.D.

Medical Service
Veterans Administration Medical Center
and
University of Kentucky College of Medicine, Lexington

BEVERLY SIELING, R.D.

Dietetic Service
Veterans Administration Medical Center
Lexington, Kentucky

Address correspondence to James W. Anderson, M.D., Medical Service, Veterans Administration Medical Center, Lexington, Kentucky 40511.

ABSTRACT

Diet is the keystone for successful management of every individual with diabetes. Traditional high-fat diets have major disadvantages; high levels of fat intake decrease sensitivity to insulin, block cellular glucose disposal, and increase serum lipids. High-carbohydrate diets increase insulin sensitivity, facilitate glucose use, and attenuate inappropriate glucose production. High-fiber diets delay and smooth out glucose absorption, increase insulin sensitivity, and lower serum lipids. Fiber-supplemented diets improve glucose metabolism over the short term and decrease insulin requirements over the long term. High-carbohydrate, high-fiber (HCF) diets dramatically lower insulin requirements of lean insulin-dependent as well as non-insulin-dependent diabetic individuals over a period of a few weeks. These diets lower serum cholesterol values by 30% and triglycerides by 14%. Long-term use of high-fiber maintenance diets sustains improvements in glucose metabolism and plasma lipid values. Different starchy foods are associated with extremely variable blood glucose responses. While potatoes providing 50 g of complex carbohydrate produce 75% of the glycemic response of 50 g of glucose, kidney beans produce only 29% as much post-meal hyperglycemia. The glycemic response to different foods may influence the development of new exchange lists for diabetes management. Normalizing blood lipids is an important goal in nutrition management. Oat-bran and beans, rich in water-soluble fiber, can lower serum cholesterol values by 20% without alterations in cholesterol or fat intake. High-fiber diets lower serum triglycerides by 60–90%. Many lines of evidence suggest that a prudent diet for most diabetic individuals should provide generous amounts of complex carbohydrate and fiber, and restrict animal fat intake.

INTRODUCTION

Nutrition guidance is critical for successful management of diabetes mellitus. Yet, recommendations regarding the carbohydrate content of the diet remain controversial. Recently, several national diabetes

50

associations recommended that the diet for most diabetic individuals should be generous in complex carbohydrate and fiber, and restricted in animal fat (1). This advice represents a departure from the traditional thinking that most diabetic individuals should moderately restrict simple and complex carbohydrate intake and consume generous amounts of fat (2). Whereas traditional diets provided approximately 40% of the energy as carbohydrate, 20% as protein, and 40% as fat, these new recommendations suggest an intake of 55–60% carbohydrate, 15–20% protein, and less than 30% fat. Many basic and clinical studies indicate that increased carbohydrate intake enhances insulin sensitivity and glucose metabolism, while increased fat intake impairs insulin sensitivity and glucose metabolism.

The role of dietary (plant) fiber in diabetes management has generated considerable interest. Recent attention has focused on the glycemic response to different foods. We will review some recent evidence regarding the effects of carbohydrate or fat intake on glucose metabolism, summarize the clinical data on fiber intake for diabetic individuals, and provide an overview of the clinical studies relating to the glycemic response to different foods. We will also briefly discuss the nutrition management of hyperlipidemias as it relates to diabetes. Finally, we will integrate these various observations and provide guidelines for a prudent diet for individuals with diabetes.

CARBOHYDRATE INTAKE AND GLUCOSE METABOLISM

Normal Individuals

High-carbohydrate, low-fat diets usually improve glucose metabolism of normal individuals (3–6). These diets tend to lower fasting plasma glucose concentrations as well as plasma glucose concentrations during oral glucose tolerance tests. Using different experimental designs, some groups (7,8) have not noted improvement of glucose metabolism with high-carbohydrate, low-fat diets. Unfortunately all of these studies (3–8) utilized liquid-formula diets containing simple sugars as the source of carbohydrate. Long-term studies (2,9) and epidemiologic studies (10) indicate that the habitual intake of diets generous in complex carbohydrate and restricted in fat is associated with better glucose tolerance than is the intake of high-fat diets.

Diabetic Individuals

High-carbohydrate, low-fat diets usually improve glucose metabolism in diabetic patients (2). After insulin became available, several groups (2,11) reported that high-carbohydrate, low-fat diets lowered insulin requirements of lean diabetic patients. Two careful studies (12,13), however, indicated that moderately high-carbohydrate, low-fiber diets did not influence glycemic control, insulin requirements, or oral hypoglycemic needs of diabetic patients. In 1976, we (14) reported that high-carbohydrate, high-fiber (HCF) diets lowered the insulin requirements of lean diabetic patients. These studies have been extended (15) and confirmed (16—19). These recent studies clearly indicate that high-carbohydrate, low-fat diets lower insulin requirements of lean insulin-dependent diabetic patients and eliminate the insulin needs of most lean non-insulin-dependent diabetic patients (20,21). With HCF diets, the lower insulin requirements are related, in part, to the high fiber content of these diets, but most of the reduction in insulin requirements is related to the high-carbohydrate and low-fat content (22). HCF diets providing 70% of energy as carbohydrate and only 12% as fat induce rapid reductions in insulin requirements; these improvements, however, can be sustained for up to eight years of outpatient follow-up with maintenance diets providing 55—60% carbohydrate and 25—30% fat (23). These recent studies clearly document that high-carbohydrate, low-fat diets offer major benefits for the management of selected individuals with diabetes.

Mechanisms

High-carbohydrate diets improve glucose metabolism by increasing the number of insulin receptors and by improving intracellular utilization of glucose. Several studies in humans (22,24,25) indicate that HCF diets increase the number of insulin receptors per cell for circulating monocytes. Based on animal studies (6), these increases in the number of insulin receptors appear related in large part to the high-carbohydrate content of these diets. High-carbohydrate diets stimulate glucose utilization in a variety of tissues (6) and increase the activities of the key enzymes involved in glycolysis. These diets stimulate glycogen synthesis and glycogen accumulation in several tissues of experimental animals. Finally, high-carbohydrate diets attenuate glucose production in the liver and decrease activities of the critical enzymes involved in gluconeogenesis (6).

FAT INTAKE AND GLUCOSE METABOLISM

In normal individuals, high-fat diets impair glucose metabolism and produce insulin resistance (26,27). The effects of high-fat diets, however, have not been as extensively documented as those of high-carbohydrate diets. High-fat diets do increase serum free fatty acid

(FFA) concentrations, which act to antagonize the action of insulin (28).

In diabetic patients, the effects of high-fat diets on insulin requirements and glucose metabolism have not been well studied. Ernst and colleagues (29) noted no differences in average blood glucose values or insulin requirements for diabetic patients fed high-fat versus high-carbohydrate diets for three weeks. The recent studies (14–18) indicating that insulin requirements fall dramatically with high-carbohydrate diets suggest that the control diets (29) providing moderate amounts of fat were sustaining a moderate insulin-resistant state.

Mechanisms

In experimental animals, high-fat diets have profound effects on glucose metabolism. Table 1 summarizes these effects. High-fat diets induce insulin resistance and impair intracellular glucose metabolism by a variety of mechanisms. The binding of insulin to insulin receptors on the surface of selected cells initiates the cascade of events triggered by insulin. High-fat diets reduce the number of insulin receptors in several types of tissue. Insulin facilitates the transport of glucose into muscle and fat cells; high-fat diets decrease glucose uptake by these cells.

Table 1. Detrimental Effects of High-Fat Diets on Glucose Metabolism[a]

Insulin receptor number—decreased for liver, muscle, and fat
Glucose uptake—decreased for muscle and fat
Glycolysis—decreased for liver, muscle, and fat
    Glucokinase activity—decreased in liver
    Hexokinase activity—decreased in muscle and fat
    Phosphofructokinase activity—decreased in liver
    Pyruvate kinase activity—decreased in liver
    Glucose-6-phosphate dehydrogenase activity—decreased in liver
Glycogen synthesis—decreased in liver and muscle
Glucose oxidation—decreased in muscle and fat
Gluconeogenesis—increased in liver
    Phosphoenolpyruvate carboxykinase activity—increased in liver

[a]Data presented or summarized elsewhere (2,6,27,28,30–33).

Insulin stimulates glycogen synthesis, glycolysis, and glucose oxidation, while high-fat diets impair all of the intracellular routes of glucose disposal.

Intracellular glycolysis, the conversion of glucose to pyruvate or lactate, is critically dependent on three key enzymes: glucokinase (or hexokinase), phosphofructokinase, and pyruvate kinase (33). While high-carbohydrate diets increase the intracellular activity of these three enzymes, high-fat diets decrease their activity. Aerobic glycolysis, also termed the pentose phosphate pathway, is critically dependent on two key enzymes: glucose-6-phosphate dehydrogenase and 6-phosphogluconate dehydrogenase. While high-carbohydrate diets increase the activity of these key enzymes, high-fat diets decrease their activity, as well as decreasing glucose oxidation to carbon dioxide and water.

A major contributor to hyperglycemia in diabetic patients is the unrestrained output of glucose by the liver. Glucose production from amino acids and lactic acid, termed gluconeogenesis, is responsible for this hyperglycemic effect. High-fat diets stimulate gluconeogenesis and, thus, directly act to raise the blood glucose concentration of normal or diabetic individuals.

High serum concentrations of free fatty acids (FFA) may be responsible for some of the adverse effects of high-fat diets on glucose metabolism. The high FFA concentrations associated with high-fat diets may act directly to reduce the number of insulin receptors of various tissues (34). The intracellular metabolism of FFA acts directly to inhibit the essential glycolytic enzyme phosphofructokinase and still further acts to stimulate gluconeogenesis (27,28).

FIBER AND GLUCOSE METABOLISM

Dietary or plant fiber has received attention from the nutrition community during the previous decade due to the hypothesis that various diseases in the Western world may be linked to fiber-depleted diets (2). Heart disease, colon disease, obesity, and diabetes are far more common among Western people than among rural populations that habitually consume high complex carbohydrate diets with large amounts of fiber. The prevalence of diabetes, for example, was almost nine times greater in a U.S. city than in East Pakistan, where the customary diet was high in fiber (10). There is more circumstantial evidence linking fiber-depleted diets to diabetes than to any other disease (2). Nevertheless, no conclusive evidence is available to clearly link any disease process to a low intake of fiber.

Definitions

Plant fibers are the portions of plant foods that are not digested in the human small intestine (35). Most fibers, except lignin, are polysaccharides which reside in the plant cell wall. Most plant fiber polysaccharides are almost completely fermented by bacteria in the colon to form short-chain fatty acids and other products such as methane, hydrogen, carbon dioxide, and water. Acetate, propionate, and butyrate—the predominant short-chain fatty acids—are almost completely absorbed into the portal vein and largely metabolized in the liver. Over 250 different fiber polysaccharides have been identified. For convenience, these fiber polysaccharides are classified as water-soluble and water-insoluble fibers. Water-soluble fibers such as gums, pectins, mucins, and other polysaccharides have major effects on glucose and cholesterol metabolism, but have little effect on fecal bulk. Dried beans, oat and barley products, and fruits are major dietary sources of water-soluble fibers. Water-insoluble fibers, such as cellulose, lignin, and cellulose-like polysaccharides (also termed hemicelluloses), have major effects on bowel function and also increase fecal bulk. Grain products, especially wheat bran, and vegetables are major dietary sources of water-insoluble fiber (35).

Glucose Metabolism in Normal Individuals

Guar gum and similar water-soluble fibers slow glucose absorption from the small intestine (36). When guar is given with glucose as part of a glucose tolerance test, the blood glucose rise is much less than when glucose alone is given. Guar-supplemented meals are followed by much lower blood glucose values than are identical meals without guar. Not only does guar decrease post-meal glycemia, it also decreases plasma insulin responses. Thus, glucose is disposed of more efficiently with less insulin secretion indicating that guar enhances insulin sensitivity. These innovative and pioneering experiments of Jenkins and colleagues (36–38) paved the way for use of guar supplements for the treatment of diabetic individuals.

Diabetes and Fiber Supplements

When guar is incorporated into standard meals of diabetic individuals, postprandial (after-meal) hyperglycemia is significantly less than after control meals without guar. After documenting these acute benefits in 1976, Jenkins and colleagues (36–38) systematically studied the short-term and long-term effects of guar supplements for insulin-treated diabetic individuals. The short-term experience indicated that guar supplements significantly decreased glucose excretion in urine. One of the disadvantages of purified guar preparations is the nausea that often accompanies guar intake. Guar powder hydrates so rapidly that it begins to gel in the mouth and esophagus and can cause unpleasant side effects. Jenkins and colleagues (38) developed a guar crispbread, resembling Melba toast, that was quite well tolerated. They noted that the long-term intake of guar crispbread improved blood glucose values and lowered insulin requirements. They reported no adverse side effects and observed no detrimental effects on mineral status (38). These studies have been confirmed by other groups (39,40). Recently a palatable form of guar in mini-tablet form (Glucotard®, Boehringer Mannheim, Germany) has been released (41). Palatable preparations of guar may offer distinct therapeutic advantages for selected patients with either insulin-dependent or non-insulin-dependent forms of diabetes.

Diabetes and High-Fiber Diets

In 1976, we (14) reported that high-carbohydrate, high-fiber diets lowered insulin requirements of lean diabetic patients. Over the next three years we carefully evaluated the effects of HCF diets on lean, insulin-treated adult diabetic men (15,20). The HCF diets used for intensive therapy in the hospital provide 70% of the energy as carbohydrate, 18% as protein, and 12% as fat, with 65–70 g of plant fiber per day. For lean adult men with insulin-dependent diabetes (Type I), these diets lower insulin requirements by 25 to 50% (Fig. 1). However, for another group of lean men treated with 25–40 units of insulin daily, intensive treatment with HCF diets eliminated their need for insulin (Fig. 1); some of these men have maintained glycemic control for up to eight years without insulin (23). Thus, HCF diets substantially lower insulin requirements for individuals with insulin-dependent (Type I) diabetes and allow management of lean non-insulin-dependent (Type II) diabetic individuals with intensive diet therapy alone. The benefits of HCF-type diets for Type I and Type II diabetic patients have been confirmed by many other groups (16–18,21,24). HCF diets not only lower insulin requirements and improve glycemic control, but they also lower average serum cholesterol concentrations by 30% and triglycerides by 14% (15,42). Our short-term experience with HCF diets mandated the evaluation of the long-term effects of HCF-type diets.

High-Fiber Diets for Long-Term Management of Diabetes

We assessed the long-term effectiveness, practicality, palatability, and safety of high-fiber diets for lean diabetic patients. We developed high-fiber maintenance diets providing 55–60% of energy as

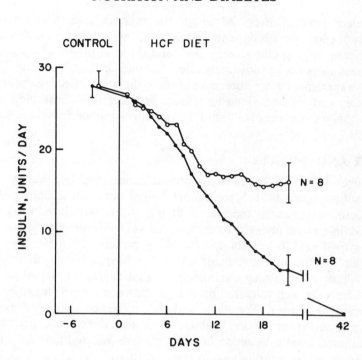

Figure 1. Response of lean, insulin-treated diabetic men to HCF diets. Insulin requirements of eight insulin-dependent (Type I) patients (open circles) were almost 50% lower on HFC than on control diets. Insulin therapy was discontinued in eight men with Type II diabetes (closed circles). Anderson, J.W. (unpublished observations).

carbohydrate, 20% as protein, 20–25% as fat, and approximately 50 g of plant fiber per day (2). These diets effectively maintain benefits obtained during hospitalization. When we discontinue insulin therapy with HCF diets, patients do not have to restart insulin injections if they closely adhere to high-fiber maintenance diets. Over an average of four years (range 2–8 years), our patients maintain satisfactory glycemic control and serum cholesterol concentrations averaging 170 mg/dl and triglycerides of 100 mg/dl (23). Our patients enjoy these high-fiber diets, and adherence is good to excellent in over 80% of the patients closely followed (43). Because these diets emphasize whole grain cereals and breads, common garden vegetables, beans, and fruits while de-emphasizing red meats, eggs, cheeses, and pastry products, we estimate that our patients' grocery bills are 20% lower than on their antecedent high-fat diets. Although our patients have more intestinal gas production (belching and flatulence), we have encountered no serious side effects. Our studies (44), and those of others (45), indicate that these diets do not adversely affect vitamin or mineral status. Thus, in our experience, high-fiber maintenance diets are effective, practical, palatable, and safe for long-term use. We feel that these diets offer major therapeutic benefits for a large proportion of individuals with diabetes.

FIBER AND OBESITY

High-fiber foods are followed by greater satiety and less hunger than are low-fiber foods (46). Since almost 75% of our adult diabetic patients are obese, we assessed the effects of high-fiber, weight-reducing diets for insulin-treated obese diabetic patients (47). We developed 800 kcal diets providing 110 g carbohydrate, 45 g protein, 20 g fat, and 32 g fiber per day for intensive treatment in the hospital. For our patients, these diets provided approximately 3 kcal/day/lb of actual weight. These diets are well tolerated by our patients and are accompanied by a minimum of hunger. For eight patients, these diets lowered average insulin doses from 59 to 1 unit/day over a three-week period; we discontinued insulin in seven of eight patients and reduced the insulin dose from 70 to 6 units/day in the eighth patient. These high-fiber, weight-reducing diets lowered blood glucose, cholesterol, and triglyceride concentrations significantly. Our patients lost 6 lbs per week on these diets. Furthermore, these diets were accompanied by minimal changes in liver function tests and serum uric acid concentrations. We feel that high-fiber, weight-reducing diets are effective and safe for intensive hospital management of poorly controlled, obese diabetic patients. Very low calorie diets (48), protein-sparing modified fasts (49), and supplemented fasting (50) are as effective in improving glycemic control and reducing insulin needs, but, in our assessment, are less safe than high-fiber, weight-reducing diets consisting of commonly available foods providing adequate protein and carbohydrate.

We are evaluating the long-term effectiveness of high-fiber weight-reducing diets for obese diabetic patients. We currently use diets providing 1200–1500 kcal daily (5 kcal/lb)—55% carbohydrate, 25% protein, and 20% fat, with approximately 50 g of fiber per day (40 g fiber/1000 kcal). With these diets some of our patients have sustained weight losses and satisfactory glycemic control without insulin therapy for over two years (J. W. Anderson, unpublished observations). Other groups (51) have reported that fiber-supplemented diets have long-term beneficial effects for obese diabetic patients. However, the effectiveness of high-fiber, weight-reducing diets or fiber-supplemented diets for obese diabetic patients has not been established. The theoretic advantages of fiber-related satiety for obese individuals remains a challenging area for further investigations.

MECHANISMS FOR FIBER ACTION

Glucose Metabolism

Plant fibers slow down glucose absorption by delaying gastric emptying, slowing the digestion of starches, and retarding the entry of glucose into absorptive cells of the small intestine (35). All of these processes decrease the rise in blood glucose concentration after a fiber-rich meal. Fiber-rich meals and high-fiber diets are associated with lower postprandial serum insulin concentrations than are observed with low-fiber meals or diets (37). Serum concentrations of other pancreatic hormones (glucagon) and gut hormones (gastric inhibitory polypeptide and enteroglucagon) are lower after high-fiber meals than after low-fiber meals. Since these hormones oppose the action of insulin, reductions in their release make individuals more sensitive to the actions of insulin (52).

Fiber intake also has indirect effects on glucose metabolism. High-fiber diets increase the number of insulin receptors, making tissues more sensitive to insulin action (22,24,25). Our studies using rat liver cells indicate that short-chain fatty acid fermentation products of fiber affect liver metabolism of glucose (53). Propionate, a three-carbon fatty acid, stimulates glucose use (glycolysis) and inhibits glucose production (gluconeogenesis) in rat liver cells. Thus, fiber intake may stimulate glucose use in liver and reduce glucose production in liver via these short-chain fatty acid products. Much further work is necessary to understand the short-term and long-term effects of fiber intake on glucose metabolism.

Lipid Metabolism

Plant fibers have substantial hypocholesterolemic effects. Water-soluble fibers, such as those contained in beans and oat products, lower serum cholesterol concentrations, while water-insoluble fibers, such as those contained in wheat bran, are not hypocholesterolemic (35). Oat-bran intake lowers serum cholesterol values by about 20% and increases fecal excretion of bile acids (54). The loss of bile acids diverts more liver cholesterol into new bile acids, and less liver cholesterol is available for secretion of cholesterol-rich lipoproteins into the blood. Our recent studies indicate that short-chain fatty acid products of fiber act to block hepatic cholesterol synthesis (53). Thus, soluble fibers may increase demands on bile acid production while decreasing the capacity of the liver to make cholesterol; these actions would obviously lower serum cholesterol concentrations.

Plant fibers also have distinct triglyceride-lowering effects (20,42). A mixture of foods containing both water-soluble and water-insoluble fibers acts to lower serum triglyceride concentrations. We do not understand how fibers lower serum triglyceride values. Currently we postulate that these two mechanisms contribute to the triglyceride-lowering effect of fibers. First, fiber intake is accompanied by lower serum insulin concentrations. Since insulin is a potent stimulus to both triglyceride synthesis in liver and very low-density lipoprotein secretion by liver, lower insulin concentrations should lower serum triglyceride concentrations. Second, fiber intake slows the absorption of fat from the intestine. By mechanisms that we do not understand, the slower and smoother delivery of fatty acids to the liver may lower serum triglyceride concentrations.

GLYCEMIC RESPONSE TO DIFFERENT FOODS

Not all carbohydrate-rich foods raise the blood glucose concentration to a similar extent when equivalent amounts of carbohydrate are fed. Simple sugars tend to raise the blood glucose more than complex carbohydrates. These well-established facts have guided nutrition counseling of diabetic individuals for decades. Recent studies, however, indicate that not all starchy foods have the same glycemic potential. Potatoes raise the blood glucose almost as much as glucose does, while beans have a minimal effect on blood glucose values. With renewed interest in the role of carbohydrate intake for diabetic individuals, the glycemic response to different complex carbohydrates is being examined. Crapo (55–57), Jenkins (58–60), O'Dea (61–63) and their colleagues have greatly extended our knowledge in this area.

Careful studies reveal surprising differences in the glycemic responses to similar foods. White bread is much more hyperglycemic than is spaghetti, while white potatoes are much more hyperglycemic than are sweet potatoes (59). Figure 2 demonstrates the different glycemic responses to bread and lentils. In studies of normal individuals, Jenkins and colleagues (59) computed the area under the blood glucose response to different foods. They termed this the "glycemic index" and used the response to glucose as the reference point, or 100%. Selected other foods rate as follows: white potatoes

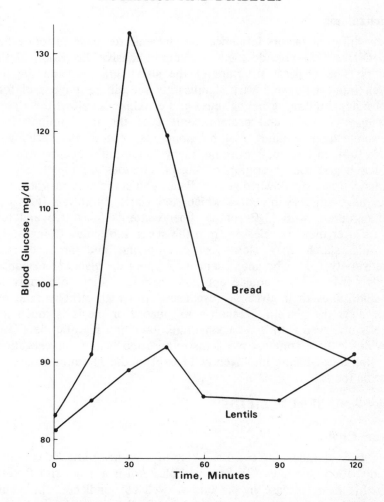

Figure 2. Glycemic response of four normal subjects to 50 g of carbohydrate from either bread or beans (from reference 59).

75%, white rice 72%, white bread 79%, All Bran cereal 51%, peas 51%, spaghetti 50%, oatmeal 49%, kidney beans 29%, and lentils 29%. These studies have important implications in the nutrition management of diabetes and may require that new exchange lists be developed.

Mechanisms

Many different factors influence the glycemic response to foods. Snow and O'Dea (62) provide the most comprehensive discussion of these factors. The physical structure of the starch granules and the fiber-starch interrelationship vary significantly for different types of foods. Processing (milling, grinding, etc.) and cooking also affect the glycemic response. The fat and protein content of the meal influences the gastrointestinal handling and hormone response to the carbohydrate foods (63). In the small intestine, many factors influence the hydrolysis of starch and the absorption of sugars. Potatoes are rapidly digested, while legumes are slowly digested. Beans and stone-ground whole wheat flour have amylase inhibitors which slow starch hydrolysis (62). Beans and oat bran, with high soluble fiber contents, may trap and retain sugars after they are released from the starch molecule. Coingestion of fat and starch may slow gastric emptying and produce insulin insensitivity (63). The antecedent meal alters the glycemic response to foods (64). The antecedent or habitual diet of individuals predetermines their glycemic responses; with high-carbohydrate, high-fiber diets the glycemic response to glucose or meals is much lower than is observed with low-carbohydrate, low-fiber, high-fat diets (1,65). Obviously these complex problems require much more investigation to propose mechanisms intelligently to explain the glycemic response to specific foods.

DIET AND SERUM LIPIDS

Serum Cholesterol

Diabetic individuals are twice as likely to have heart attacks as matched nondiabetic individuals (2). Serum cholesterol is a major risk factor for ischemic heart disease in diabetic as well as nondiabetic individuals. One goal of nutrition management of diabetic individuals is to minimize the risks for atherosclerosis by maintaining healthy or safe serum cholesterol concentrations. Healthy or safe ranges for serum cholesterol are not established, but we like to maintain serum cholesterol values below 200 mg/dl for our patients; we consider a healthy cholesterol to be 140 mg/dl plus the age of the patient. Many nutrition maneuvers lower serum cholesterol values; low-cholesterol, low-fat diets are moderately effective (42). Our HCF diets lower serum cholesterol concentrations by 30% (15,42). Oat bran (54) or bean supplements have significant cholesterol-lowering properties (35). These soluble-fiber rich foods can lower serum cholesterol concentrations of hypercholesterolemic men by 20% without changes in fat or cholesterol intake. When hypercholesterolemic individuals use oat-bran supplements, 50 g/day or four oat-bran muffins, serum cholesterol values are sustained at 20% below initial values for up to two years (66). Oat-bran supplemented diets selectively lower atherogenic low-density lipoprotein cholesterol concentrations while raising protective high-density lipoprotein cholesterol concentrations in serum.

By following high-fiber maintenance diets (55% carbohydrate, 20% protein, 25% fat, and 50 g fiber/day) our diabetic patients maintain "healthy" serum cholesterol concentrations averaging 170 mg/dl (23). When diabetic or nondiabetic individuals have hypercholesterolemia, we advise them to incorporate more oat bran and beans into their diet. This approach has been very effective for patients with mild or moderate hypercholesterolemia (66).

Serum Triglycerides

Hypertriglyceridemia is a risk factor for atherosclerosis in diabetic patients. We attempt to maintain fasting serum triglyceride concentrations below 200 mg/dl for our diabetic patients. HCF diets lower serum triglyceride concentrations dramatically for hypertriglyceridemic patients (20). We evaluated short-term and long-term effects of high-fiber diets for 10 men with fasting serum triglyceride concentrations exceeding 1000 mg/dl. Initial serum triglyceride values were approximately 2500 mg/dl; HCF diets in the hospital lowered values to approximately 500 mg/dl. With long-term adherence to high-fiber maintenance diets, average triglyceride values were 250 mg/dl (J.W. Anderson, unpublished observations). Thus HCF diets (70% carbohydrate) and high-fiber maintenance diets (55% carbohydrate) lower average fasting serum triglyceride concentrations in both diabetic and hypertriglyceridemic individuals. Our studies support previous reports (5,67—69) that diets generous in complex carbohydrate and fiber and restricted in fat and cholesterol are effective for the initial nutrition management of most individuals with hyperlipidemia.

A PRUDENT DIET

We developed high-fiber maintenance diets for the long-term management of diabetic individuals. These diets provide 55—60% of the energy as carbohydrate, 20% as protein, and 20—25% as fat, less than 200 mg of cholesterol per day, and 50 g of plant fiber daily (25 g/1000 kcal). These diets lower insulin requirements, improve glycemic control, and lower serum cholesterol and triglyceride concentrations. Our patients enjoy these diets and closely adhere to them. We have not encountered undesirable side-effects and have not detected vitamin or mineral deficiencies by measurement of serum levels. These high-fiber maintenance diets appear suitable for management of many adults with diabetes.

Our nutrition plan for diabetic individuals coincides with the current recommendations of the American Diabetes Association and several other national diabetes associations (1). The American Heart Association (70) recently recommended similar nutrition principles as a prudent approach to reduce the risk for atherosclerosis. All of these recommendations can be followed without drastic changes in eating habits. A typical breakfast provides a serving of fruit or juice, a whole grain cereal with skim or low-fat milk, whole wheat toast, and margarine. A representative noon meal provides tomato juice, a turkey sandwich with lettuce and tomato, a marinated bean salad, and fruit. An evening meal could consist of a spinach-mushroom salad with low-fat dressing, lentil soup, baked fish, baked potato, green beans, pickled beets, bran muffins, margarine, and a fruit dessert. All of these foods are commonly used by Americans and available at most grocery stores. This nutrition plan may offer benefits for adults at risk for diabetes, ischemic heart disease, hypertension (71), or obesity.

REFERENCES

1. R. Arky, J. Wylie-Rosett, and B. El-Beheri, Examination of current dietary recommendations for individuals with diabetes mellitus. *Diabetes Care* 5, 59 (1982).
2. J. W. Anderson, The role of dietary carbohydrate and fiber in the control of diabetes. *Adv. Intern. Med.* 26, 67 (1981).
3. J. D. Brunzell, R. L. Lerner, W. R. Hazzard, D. Porte, Jr., and E. L. Bierman, Improved glucose tolerance with high carbohydrate feeding in mild diabetes. *N. Engl. J. Med.* 284, 521 (1971).
4. J. W. Anderson, R. E. Herman, and R. H. Herman, Effect of high sucrose diets on glucose tolerance of normal men. *Am. J. Clin. Nutr.* 26, 600 (1973).
5. B. Schellenberg, P. Oster, G. Vogel, C. C. Hueck, and G. Schlierf, 24-hour patterns of blood sugar, plasma insulin and free fatty acids in patients with primary endogenous hyperlipoproteinemia on isocaloric diets containing 30, 43, and 79% carbohydrates. *Nutr. Med.* 23, 316 (1979).
6. J. W. Anderson, High carbohydrate diet effects on glucose and triglyceride metabolism of normal and diabetic men. In S. Reiser, ed. *Metabolic Effects of Utilizable Dietary Carbohydrates*, Marcel Dekker, New York, 1982.

7. J.W. Farquhar, A. Frank, and R.C. Gross, Glucose, insulin and triglyceride response to high and low carbohydrate diets in man. *J. Clin. Invest.* **45**, 1648 (1966).

8. G.M. Reaven and J.M. Olefsky, Increased plasma glucose and insulin responses to high-carbohydrate feedings in normal subjects. *J. Clin. Endo. Metab.* **38**, 151 (1974).

9. E. Farinaro, J. Stamler, M. Upton, L. Monjonnier, Y. Hall, D. Moss, and D.M. Berkson, Long term effect of diet in the Chicago Coronary Prevention Evaluation Program. *Ann. Intern. Med.* **86**, 147 (1977).

10. K.M. West and J.M. Kalbfleisch, Influence of nutritional factors on prevalence of diabetes. *Diabetes* **20**, 99 (1971).

11. I.M. Rabinowitch, Effects of the high carbohydrate—low calorie diet on carbohydrate tolerance in diabetes mellitus. *Can. Med. Assoc. J.* **33**, 136 (1935).

12. D.B. Stone and W.E. Connor, The prolonged effects of a low cholesterol high carbohydrate diet on the serum lipids in diabetic patients. *Diabetes* **12**, 127 (1963).

13. R.L. Weinsier, A. Seeman, G. Herrera, J. Assal, J.S. Soeldner, and R.E. Gleason, High and low carbohydrate diets in diabetes mellitus. *Ann. Intern. Med.* **80**, 332 (1974).

14. T.G. Kiehm, J.W. Anderson, and K. Ward, Beneficial effects of a high carbohydrate, high fiber diet on hyperglycemic diabetic men. *Am. J. Clin. Nutr.* **29**, 895 (1976).

15. J.W. Anderson and K. Ward, High carbohydrate, high fiber diets for insulin-treated men with diabetes mellitus. *Am. J. Clin. Nutr.* **32**, 2312 (1979).

16. R.W. Simpson, J.I. Mann, J. Eaton, R.D. Carter, and T.D.R. Hockaday, High carbohydrate diets and insulin-dependent diabetics. *Br. Med. J.* **2**, 523 (1979).

17. A.L. Kinmonth, R.M. Angus, P.A. Jenkins, M.A. Smith, and J.D. Baum, Whole foods and increased dietary fibre improve blood glucose control in diabetic children. *Arch. Dis. Childhood* **57**, 187 (1982).

18. D. Ney, D.R. Hollingsworth, and L. Cousins, Decreased insulin requirement and improved control of diabetes in pregnant women given a high-carbohydrate, high-fiber, low-fat diet. *Diabetes Care* **5**, 529 (1982).

19. M.R. Taskinen, E.A. Nikkila, and A. Ollus, Serum lipids and lipoproteins in insulin-dependent diabetic subjects during high-carbohydrate, high-fiber diet. *Diabetes Care* **6**, 224 (1983).

20. J.W. Anderson, High-fiber diets in diabetes and hypertriglyceridemia. *Can. Med. Assoc. J.* **123**, 975 (1980).

21. R.J. Barnard, M.R. Massey, S. Cherny, L.T. O'Brien, and N. Pritikin, Long-term use of a high-complex-carbohydrate, high-fiber, low-fat diet in the treatment of NIDDM patients. *Diabetes Care* **6**, 268 (1983).

22. J.W. Anderson, High carbohydrate, high fiber diets for patients with diabetes. *Treatment of Early Diabetes* **99**, 263 (1979).

23.   J. W. Anderson and K. Ward, Long-term effects of high-carbohydrate, high-fiber diets on glucose and lipid metabolism: A preliminary report on patients with diabetes. *Diabetes Care* 1, 77 (1978).

24.   O. Pedersen, E. Hollund, H. O. Lindskov, P. Helms, N. S. Sorensen, and J. Ditzel, Increased insulin receptor binding to monocytes from insulin-dependent diabetic patients after a low-fat, high-starch, high-fiber diet. *Diabetes Care* 5, 284 (1982).

25.   G. M. Ward, R. W. Simpson, H. C. R. Simpson, B. A. Naylor, J. I. Mann, and R. C. Turner, Insulin receptor binding increased by high carbohydrate low fat diet in non-insulin-dependent diabetics. *Eur. J. Clin. Inv.* 12, 93 (1982).

26.   H. P. Himswroth, The physiological activation of insulin. *Clin. Sci.* 1, 1 (1933).

27.   C. N. Hales and R. Randle, Effects of low-carbohydrate diet and diabetes mellitus on plasma concentrations of glucose, nonesterified free fatty acids, and insulin during oral glucose tolerance tests. *Lancet* 1, 790 (1963).

28.   N. B. Ruderman, C. J. Toews, and E. Shafrir, Free fatty acids in glucose homeostasis. *Arch. Intern. Med.* 123, 299 (1969).

29.   T. Ernest, B. Hallgren, and A. Svanborg, Short-term study of effect of different isocaloric diets in diabetes. *Metabolism* 11, 912 (1962).

30.   J. M. Olefsky and M. Saekow, The effects of dietary carbohydrate content on insulin binding and glucose metabolism in isolated rat adipocytes. *Endocrinology* 103, 2252 (1978).

31.   P. J. Hissin, E. Karnieli, I. A. Simpson, L. B. Salans, and S. W. Cushman, A possible mechanism of insulin resistance in the rat adipose cell with high-fat/low-carbohydrate feeding. *Diabetes* 31, 589 (1982).

32.   M. L. Grundleger and S. W. Thenen, Decreased insulin binding, glucose transport and glucose metabolism in soleus muscle of rats fed a high fat diet. *Diabetes* 31, 232 (1982).

33.   J. W. Anderson and R. H. Herman, Effects of carbohydrate restriction on glucose tolerance of normal men, reactive hypoglycemic and diabetic patients. *Am. J. Clin. Nutr.* 28, 748 (1975).

34.   C. Grunfeld, K. L. Baird, and C. R. Kahn, Maintenance of 3T3-L1 cells in culture media containing saturated fatty acids decreases insulin binding and insulin action. *Biochem. Biophys. Res. Commun.* 103, 219 (1981).

35.   J. W. Anderson and W. L. Chen, Plant fiber: Carbohydrate and lipid metabolism. *Am. J. Clin. Nutr.* 32, 346 (1979).

36.   D. J. A. Jenkins, W. M. S. Wolever, A. R. Leeds, M. A. Gassull, P. Haisman, J. Dilawari, D. V. Goff, G. L. Metz, and K. G. M. M. Alberti, Dietary fibres, fibre analogues, and glucose tolerance: Importance of viscosity. *Br. Med. J.* 1, 1392 (1978).

37.   D. J. A. Jenkins, T. M. S. Wolever, R. Haworth, A. R. Leeds, and T. D. R. Hockaday, Guar gum in diabetes. *Lancet* 2, 1086 (1976).

38.   D. J. A. Jenkins, T. M. S. Wolever, R. H. Taylor, D. Reynolds, R. Nineham, and T. D. Hockaday, Diabetic glucose control, lipids, and trace

elements on long-term guar. *Br. Med. J.* **1**, 1353 (1980).

39. A. Aro, M. Uusitupa, E. Voutilainen, K. Hersio, T. Korhonen, and O. Siitonen, Improved diabetic control and hypocholesterolemic effect induced by long-term dietary supplementation with guar gum in Type 2 (insulin-independent) diabetes. *Diabetologia* **21**, 29 (1981).

40. K. Johansen, Decreased urinary glucose excretion and plasma cholesterol level in non-insulin-dependent diabetic patients with guar. *Diabetes Metab.* **4**, 87 (1981).

41. D. Moor, K. Huth, C. Brauning, and J. Vollmar, Untersuchungen über die wirkung von guargranulat bei stationären patienten mit manifestem diabetes mellitus. *Akt. Endokr. Stoffwe. Chsel.* **1**, 190 (1980).

42. J. W. Anderson, W. L. Chen, and B. Sieling, Hypolipidemic effects of high-carbohydrate, high-fiber diets. *Metabolism* **29**, 551 (1980).

43. L. Story, J. W. Anderson, B. Sieling, and W. Chen, High-carbohydrate, high-fiber diets for lean insulin-treated diabetic patients. *Diabetes* **31**, 58A (1982).

44. J. W. Anderson, S. K. Ferguson, D. Karounos, L. O'Malley, B. Sieling, and W. L. Chen, Mineral and vitamin status on high-fiber diets: Long-term studies of diabetic patients. *Diabetes Care* **3**, 38 (1980).

45. J. Rattan, N. Levin, E. Graff, N. Weizer, and T. Gilat, A high fiber diet does not cause mineral and nutrient deficiencies. *J. Clin. Gastroent.* **3**, 389 (1981).

46. G. B. Haber, K. W. Heaton, D. Murphy, and L. F. Burroughs, Depletion and disruption of dietary fibre, effects on satiety, plasma-glucose and serum insulin. *Lancet* **2**, 679 (1977).

47. J. W. Anderson and B. Sieling, High fiber diets for obese diabetic patients. *Obesity Bariat. Med.* **9**, 109 (1980).

48. A. N. Howard, The historical development, efficacy and safety of very-low-calorie diets. *Int. J. Obesity* **5**, 1 (1981).

49. B. R. Bistrain, G. L. Blackburn, J. P. Flatt, J. Sizer, N. S. Scrimshaw, and M. Sherman, Nitrogen metabolism and insulin requirements in obese diabetic adults in a protein-sparing modified fast. *Diabetes* **25**, 494 (1976).

50. S. M. Genuth, Supplemented fasting in the treatment of obesity and diabetes. *Am. J. Clin. Nutr.* **32**, 2579 (1979).

51. T. K. Ray, K. M. Mansell, L. C. Knight, L. S. Malmud, O. E. Owen, and G. Boden, Long-term effects of dietary fiber on glucose tolerance and gastric emptying in noninsulin dependent diabetic patients. *Am. J. Clin, Nutr.* **37**, 376 (1983).

52. J. W. Anderson, Dietary fiber and diabetes. In G. V. Vahouny, ed., *Dietary Fiber*, Plenum, New York, 1982.

53. J. W. Anderson and S. R. Bridges, Plant-fiber metabolites alter hepatic glucose and lipid metabolism. *Diabetes* **30**, 133A (1981).

54. R. W. Kirby, J. W. Anderson, B. Sieling, E. D. Rees, W. L. Chen, R. E. Miller, and R. M. Kay, Oat-bran selectively lowers serum low density lipoprotein cholesterol concentrations of hypercholesterolemic men. *Am. J. Clin. Nutr.* **34**, 824 (1981).

55. P. A. Crapo, G. Reaven, and J. Olefsky, Plasma glucose and insulin responses to orally administered simple and complex carbohydrates. *Diabetes* 25, 741 (1976).

56. P. A. Crapo, G. Reaven, and J. Olefsky, Post-prandial plasma-glucose and insulin responses to different complex carbohydrates. *Diabetes* 26, 1178 (1977).

57. P. A. Crapo, O. G. Kolterman, N. Waldeck, G. M. Reaven, and J. M. Olefsky, Postprandial hormonal responses to different types of complex carbohydrates in individuals with impaired glucose tolerance. *Am. J. Clin. Nutr.* 33, 1723 (1980).

58. D. J. A. Jenkins, T. M. S. Wolever, R. H. Taylor, H. M. Barker, and H. Fielden, Exceptionally low blood glucose response to dried beans: Comparison with other carbohydrate foods. *Br. Med. J.* 30, 578 (1980).

59. D. J. A. Jenkins, D. M. Thomas, M. S. Wolever, R. H. Taylor, H. Barker, H. Fielden, J. M. Baldwin, A. C. Bowling, H. C. Newman, A. L. Jenkins, and D. V. Goff, Glycemic index of foods: A physiological basis for carbohydrate exchange. *Am. J. Clin. Nutr.* 34, 362 (1981).

60. D. J. A. Jenkins, H. Ghafari, T. M. S. Wolever, R. H. Taylor, A. L. Jenkins, H. M. Barker, H. Fielden, and A. C. Bowling, Relationship between rate of digestion of foods and postprandial glycaemia. *Diabetologia* 22, 450 (1982).

61. K. O'Dea, P. Nestel, and L. Antonoff, Physical factors influencing postprandial glucose and insulin responses to starch. *Am. J. Clin. Nutr.* 33, 760 (1980).

62. P. Snow and K. O'Dea, Factors affecting the rate of hydrolysis of starch in food. *Am. J. Clin. Nutr.* 34, 2721 (1981).

63. G. Collier and K. O'Dea, Effect of physical form of carbohydrate on the postprandial glucose, insulin, and gastric inhibitory polypeptide responses in Type 2 diabetes. *Am. J. Clin. Nutr.* 36, 10 (1982).

64. D. J. A. Jenkins and T. M. S. Wolever, Slow release dietary carbohydrate improves second meal tolerance. *Am. J. Clin. Nutr.* 35, 1339 (1982).

65. A. R. P. Walker, Crude fiber, bowel motility, and the pattern of the diet. *S. African Med. J.* 35, 114 (1961).

66. J. W. Anderson, L. Story, B. Sieling, and W. Chen, Hypocholesterolemic effects of plant fiber: Short-term and long-term effects of oat bran or beans. *Clin. Res.* 29, 754A (1981).

67. W. E. Connor and S. L. Connor, The alternative American diet. *Adv. Exp. Biol. Med.* 82, 843 (1977).

68. D. Sommariva, L. Scotti, and A. Fasoli, Low-fat diet vs. low-carbohydrate diet in the treatment of type IV hyperlipoproteinaemia. *Atherosclerosis* 29, 43 (1978).

69. S. Tabaqchali, A. Chait, R. Harrison, and B. Lewis, Experience with a simplified scheme of treatment of hyperlipidemia. *Br. J. Med.* 3, 337 (1974).

70. S. M. Grundy, Rationale of the diet—heart statement of the American Heart Association. *Circulation* 65, 839A (1982).

71. J.W. Anderson, Plant fiber and blood pressure. *Ann. Intern. Med.* **98**, 842 (1983).

ADDITIONAL RECENT REFERENCES

72. J.P. Bantle, D.C. Laine, G.W. Castle, et al., Postprandial glucose and insulin responses to meals containing different carbohydrates in normal and diabetic subjects. *N. Engl. J. Med.* **309**, 7 (1983).
73. P.A. Crapo and J.M. Olefsky, Food fallacies and blood sugar. *N. Engl. J. Med.* **309**, 44 (1983).
74. G. Kolata, Dietary dogma disproved. *Science* **220**, 487 (1983).
75. F.Q. Nuttall, A.D. Mooradian, R. DeMarais, et al., The glycemic effect of different meals approximately isocaloric and similar in protein, carbohydrate, and fat content as calculated using the ADA exchange lists. *Diabetes Care* **6**, 432 (1983).
76. D.J.A. Jenkins, T.M.S. Wolever, A.L. Jenkins, et al., The glycaemic index of foods tested in diabetic patients. A new basis for carbohydrate exchange favouring the use of legumes. *Diabetologia* **24**, 257 (1983).
77. A.M. Coulston, G.C. Liu, and G.M. Reaven, Plasma glucose, insulin and lipid responses to high carbohydrate low fat diets in normal humans. *Metabolism* **32**, 52 (1983).
78. R.B. Frazier, F.A. Ford, and R.D.G. Milner, A controlled trial of a high dietary fibre intake in pregnancy—Effect on plasma glucose and insulin levels. *Diabetologia* **25**, 238 (1983).
79. E. Hjollund, O. Pedersen, B. Richelsen, et al., Increased insulin binding to adipocytes and monocytes and increased insulin sensitivity to glucose transport and metabolism in adipocytes from non-insulin dependent diabetics after á low-fat/high-starch/high-fiber diet. *Metabolism* **32**, 1067 (1983).
80. A.N. Lindsay, S. Hardy, L. Jarrett, and M.L. Rallison, High-carbohydrate, high-fiber diet in children with Type I diabetes mellitus. *Diabetes Care* **7**, 63 (1984).
81. B. Karlstrom, B. Vessby, N.-G. Asp, et al., Effects of an increased content of cereal fibre in the diet of type 2 (non-insulin-dependent) diabetic patients. *Diabetologia* **26**, 272 (1984).
82. G. Riccardi, A. Rivellese, D. Pacioni, et al., Separate influence of dietary carbohydrate and fibre on the metabolic control of diabetes. *Diabetologia* **26**, 116 (1984).
83. N.A. Blackburn, J.S. Redfern, H. Jarjis, et al., The mechanism of action of guar gum in improving glucose tolerance in man. *Clin. Sci.* **66**, 329 (1984).
84. D.J.A. Jenkins, T.M.S. Wolever, A.L. Jenkins, et al., The glycemic response to carbohydrate foods. *Lancet* (in press).

4
Nutrition and Inborn Errors of Metabolism

MARGARET A. WALLEN
Department of Genetics
University of California, Berkeley

SEYMOUR PACKMAN, M.D.
Division of Genetics
Department of Pediatrics
University of California, San Francisco

Present address of Ms. Wallen is Neurosciences Training Program, University of Wisconsin, Madison, Wisconsin 53706.
Address correspondence to Seymour Packman, M.D., Division of Genetics, Department of Pediatrics, University of California, San Francisco, California 94143.

ABSTRACT

The presymptomatic treatment of inborn errors of metabolism has benefited from the systematic application of nutritional principles and strategies of nutritional intervention. The therapeutic repertory includes: the administration of pharmacologic doses of vitamins in selected disorders, the restriction of dietary precursors of toxic metabolites, and the replacement of deficient reaction products. Of particular note is the extension of such approaches in prenatal treatment of inherited metabolic disorders. Examples are discussed, with emphasis on the rational derivation of specific treatment protocols, based on disease mechanisms and on advances in nutritional sciences.

INTRODUCTION

In this country, approximately 4% of individuals born each year have a genetic or partly genetic disorder (1). Inherited metabolic diseases contribute significantly to this total. Although individually rare, the aggregate incidence of inborn errors is relatively high, and may be significantly greater than 1/1000 newborns (2,3).

Given the significant burden of inherited disorders in general, and inborn errors of metabolism in particular, it is not surprising that recent emphasis has been on treatment and on prevention of morbidity and mortality. Treatment approaches to a variety of inborn errors have been systematized in recent work (2,4,5), and many such conditions may now be viewed by practitioners as treatable disorders. Successful therapeutic protocols have been based on an understanding of fundamental pathophysiology and disease mechanisms, and have benefited from refinements in the use of special diets in the management of inborn errors of intermediary metabolism (6). Such increasing application of nutritional principles and nutritional intervention in inherited metabolic diseases has resulted in a true symbiosis between the fields of human biochemical genetics and nutrition.

Inborn errors of metabolism are single gene disorders most often inherited as autosomal recessive traits. The diseases are the result of defective processing, disposition, or transport of small molecules such as amino acids, fatty acids, metals, or sugars. This definition reflects the pioneering concepts introduced by Sir Archibald Garrod in 1908 (7). Garrod postulated that metabolic disorders were inherited biochemical blocks in normal metabolic pathways. In this construct, reaction steps in a given intracellular metabolic sequence—as well as transport of metabolites across morphologic barriers—are mediated by proteins, and are genetically determined. Inherited disorders of the sequence may exist when there is an insufficient quantity of, or aberrant structure and function of, the proteins mediating the various steps.

Specific approaches to therapy can be directly derived from considerations of potential sources of toxicity in metabolic disorders. For example, if conversion of a substrate to a product is inadequate, the resultant dearth of product may cause disease manifestations. Alternatively, a block in a reaction step may result in an intracellular/extracellular accumulation of a substrate which may be toxic and cause disease. Further, accumulation of a given substrate may result in increased flux through an otherwise minor pathway, raising to toxic concentrations an otherwise minor metabolite. Similar consequences obtain if the block is at a transport step.

Such considerations can be used to derive general approaches to therapy. In some instances, the therapeutic exigency is the replacement of a product that is not being synthesized. Examples include administration of clotting factors in hemophilias, replacement of thyroid hormone in inherited disorders of thyroid hormonogenesis, and provision of neuroactive agents in disorders of biopterin metabolism. In other instances, it may be possible to provide an antagonist to eliminate or otherwise detoxify offending accumulated metabolites. An example is the use of penicillamine as a copper chelator in Wilson's disease. That same drug is also used to increase the solubility of urinary cystine, thereby preventing urolithiasis in children and adults with cystinuria.

Therapeutic efforts in inborn errors are often directed towards a reduction in concentration of a precursor of a defective reaction step. This approach is valid whether toxicity is due directly to a proximately accumulating reactant or to derivatives thereof, and presently constitutes a major therapeutic effort of human biochemical geneticists and clinical nutritionists. Such reduction in metabolite concentration may be achieved by dietary restriction of specific precursors or general restriction of the intake of a class of nutrient. Examples include phenylalanine restriction in classical phenylketonuria, galactose restriction in the galactosemias, and protein restriction in urea cycle defects. (The urea cycle disorders are prototypes for quite innovative treatment approaches exploiting alternative reaction pathways for removal of endogenously produced precursor nitrogen (8).)

VITAMIN-RESPONSIVE DISORDERS

Vitamin-responsive or vitamin-dependent disease constitutes a category of inborn errors in which treatment has been especially successful (9). Such disorders respond to vitamins administered in pharmacologic doses (up to 1000 times the Recommended Dietary Allowance), or by a nonphysiologic route. The basis for such successful therapeutic responses resides in the notion that vitamins have specific chemical roles, and perform these roles bound to enzymes. For example, normal catalysis in a given reaction step may require the presence and precise covalent binding to the enzyme of a cofactor (coenzyme) such as pyridoxine, cobalamin, or biotin. Failure to achieve such linkage of coenzyme to the enzyme protein (apoenzyme) will produce manifestations interpreted clinically as a disorder of that reaction step.

Vitamins are themselves small molecules, and must be absorbed, transported to and into cells, reach the appropriate cell compartment, and perhaps be converted to other chemical forms prior to attachment to the apoenzyme protein. The processing of vitamins as small molecules is, therefore, not unlike that of metabolites such as amino acids, monosaccharides, or fatty acids. There is a possibility of specificity at each processing step, with mediation of that step by a specific protein. One can anticipate that an inborn error of metabolism may affect one of these steps for a given vitamin, or may affect an apoenzyme protein so that the cofactor is poorly bound. In either instance, the end result is defective catalysis by the vitamin-dependent enzyme.

If there is residual activity of a protein mediating a reaction in vitamin processing or transport, then there exists the possibility of overcoming the block by achieving a very high concentration of the vitamin at the intracellular reaction site. For example, in the instance of the interconversion of a vitamin from one chemical form to the final coenzyme form, the presentation to a reaction system of very high concentrations of precursor vitamin may result in the formation of enough product (i.e., the coenzyme form of the vitamin) to yield a physiologically satisfactory result. In clinical practice, this is done by administering pharmacologic doses of the specific vitamin.

Cobalamin (Vitamin B-12)

An important example of genetic disorders characterized by aberrant conversions to final coenzyme form are the cobalamin-responsive methylmalonic acidemias (10–12). The vitamin hydroxocobalamin must be converted to the active coenzymes, 5'-deoxyadenosylcobalamin and methylcobalamin. The enzymatic reactions dependent on these cofactors are methylmalonyl CoA mutase and N^5-methyltetrahydrofolate-homocysteine methyltransferase, respectively. The conversion of hydroxocobalamin to 5'-deoxyadenosylcobalamin requires at least two reductase steps and a deoxyadenosyl transferase reaction. Failure to achieve such a conversion to coenzyme leads to defective function of the mutase enzyme, with failure to convert L-methylmalonyl CoA to succinyl CoA (11). Clinical consequences include protein intolerance, failure to thrive, episodic ketoacidosis, and neurologic abnormalities, with death in severe, untreated cases (11).

A number of such patients are chemically and clinically responsive to very high doses of cobalamin. In seminal and representative studies performed on a boy with a defect in the synthesis of 5'-deoxyadenosylcobalamin (10,11), the excessive excretion of methylmalonic acid fell dramatically with daily intramuscular injections of 1 mg of cyanocobalamin. Urinary methylmalonate returned to pre-treatment levels after the injections ceased. Treatment with smaller quantities of cyanocobalamin (0.05–0.24 mg/day) did not effect a reduction in methylmalonate excretion (10,11).

Several important points are illustrated by these early and most critical investigations. First is the requirement of pharmacologic doses of the cofactor to produce a therapeutic response (1 mg/day, compared with the Recommended Dietary Allowance of 0.003 mg/day). Further, whether or not the precise defect in the reaction mechanism is known, it is desirable to demonstrate a reproducible improvement in specifically aberrant clinical chemistries, so as to identify patients who are candidates for such therapeutic approaches. Finally, the ultimate designation of "responsiveness" must be derived from observations of clinical efficacy of therapy, rather than from measurements of reaction precursors or products. This is especially so in the face of our frequent inability to do more than speculate and indirectly comment on the actual mechanisms of toxicity in inborn errors (12).

Pyridoxine

The most prevalent form of homocystinuria is due to a deficiency of cystathionine-β-synthase activity, a key step in the transsulfuration pathway in which methionine is converted to cysteine (13). Clinical manifestations variably include arachnodactyly, osteoporosis, thin skin, kyphoscoliosis, thromboembolic phenomena, dislocated lenses, and mental retardation (14). About half of the patients respond to pharmacologic doses of pyridoxine (up to 1200 mg/day) (15). Vitamin responsiveness in pyridoxine-responsive cystathionine-β-synthase deficiency is not due to aberrant conversion of pyridoxine to the active cofactor, pyridoxal phosphate. Rather, the fundamental lesion resides in structural defects of the apoenzyme protein, causing impaired apoenzyme-coenzyme interaction (15,16). In at least some responsive patients, it appears that the levels to which intracellular pyridoxal phosphate concentrations can be raised by pyridoxine administration to the patient are sufficient to overcome the defective binding of pyridoxal phosphate by the apoenzyme (16).

Biotin

We herein consider the consequences of another kind of defect in the covalent bonding of cofactor to apoenzyme to form functional holoenzyme. In the case of biotin-dependent carboxylases, that covalent linkage is accomplished in an ATP- and Mg-dependent reaction catalyzed by holocarboxylase synthetase (17,18). Recently, in one category of biotin-dependent inborn errors, the underlying biochemical lesion has been identified as an abnormal holocarboxylase synthetase, with an elevated $K_{m\text{(biotin)}}$ and a decreased V_{max} (19–21).

Such patients frequently (22–27), but not invariably (28,29), present with congenital lactic acidosis of variable severity, and have been designated as neonatal-onset or type 1 (29) biotin-responsive multiple carboxylase deficiency. In these patients, a characteristic organic aciduria reflects *in vivo* functional deficiency of three mitochondrial carboxylases: propionyl CoA carboxylase, 3-methylcrotonyl CoA carboxylase, and pyruvate carboxylase. These enzymes catalyze reactions in the intermediary metabolism of carbohydrates, fatty acids, and amino acids. Rapid reversal of neurologic dysfunction, and improvement of organic aciduria (lactic acid, 3-hydroxypropionic acid, methylcitric acid, and 3-methylcrotonylglycine) has followed the oral or parenteral administration of pharmacologic doses of biotin (22–27). Pedigree data are consistent with autosomal recessive inheritance (21).

The extraordinary clinical biotin dependence of such patients is reflected in the exquisite sensitivity to biotin deprivation on the part of cultured skin fibroblasts derived from children with type 1 multiple carboxylase deficiency (22,26,30–34). In such studies, the cells of probands exhibit reduced specific activities of propionyl CoA carboxylase, pyruvate carboxylase, and 3-methylcrotonyl CoA carboxylase following growth under conditions of restricted biotin availability to the fibroblasts.

The rapid clinical response to biotin administration is also reflected in the behavior of fibroblast carboxylase activity in type 1 disease cells. Restoration of mitochondrial (and cytosolic (29)) carboxylase activities can rapidly be achieved following transfer of biotin-depleted cells to a culture medium containing high biotin concentrations (30–34).

Our group has had the opportunity to study in detail the clinical course and response to therapy in a child (22) with type 1 multiple carboxylase deficiency. In the parents' subsequent pregnancy, advantage was taken of the clinical biotin responsiveness and of the biochemical expression of the neonatal-onset mutation in fibroblasts to diagnose and treat prenatally a fetus with this form of multiple carboxylase deficiency. The objectives of such prenatal therapy were to produce high serum and tissue biotin levels in the fetus and newborn child, in order to prevent possible prenatal neurological damage and severe ketoacidosis in the perinatal period.

The prenatal diagnosis was established in two ways, from material obtained at amniocentesis at 17 weeks gestation. First, it was determined that amniotic-fluid methylcitrate was significantly elevated (21,35). Second, amniotic fluid cell carboxylase specific activities were shown to be sensitive to biotin deprivation—a response identical to that of the proband's fibroblasts (21,31).On the basis of these data, the fetus was considered to be affected, and the mother was started on 10 mg/day of oral biotin at 23½ weeks' gestation—well past the period of major organogenesis and teratogenicity risk (36). This dose schedule resulted in a 21-fold to 242-fold increase in serum biotin levels without apparent ill effect on the mother (21).

At birth, cord-blood biotin concentration was 34 times normal (21,37), and this magnitude of elevation was maintained without further supplementation during the neonatal period. Physical examinations and clinical chemistries were entirely normal, in contrast to the severely disordered perinatal course of the proband (22). Following discharge on 40 mg oral biotin per day and no dietary restrictions, growth and development have been normal to age 2¼ years. The biotin given during pregnancy was clearly adequate to elevate the baby's serum levels significantly. Further, the high serum (and, presumably, tissue) biotin concentration was successfully protective in the perinatal period.

A second form of biotin-responsive multiple carboxylase deficiency generally comes to medical attention after the newborn period, and has been accordingly termed the infantile-onset form or type 2 disease

(29,38—42). In addition to the acute clinical and chemical aberrations noted for type 1 multiple carboxylase deficiency, children with infantile-onset disease exhibit manifestations similar in some respects to the findings in human biotin deficiency (43): skin rash, keratoconjunctivitis and alopecia, immunodeficiency with mucocutaneous candidiasis, and cerebellar ataxia and developmental delay.

Type 2 multiple carboxylase deficiency is not expressed in fibroblasts, as measured by biotin dependence of carboxylases following manipulation of biotin availability to cells. However, deficient serum biotinidase activity has recently been described in a number of such patients (44). It has been proposed that the basic defect may reside in the inability of such patients to recycle biotin from endogenous biocytin (44). Should the absence of this activity prove to be a reliable marker in a cell type that can be obtained from the fetus, then prenatal diagnosis of this second form of multiple carboxylase deficiency should eventually be feasible.

The responsiveness of an inborn error of metabolism to pharmocologic doses of water-soluble vitamins has been applied in at least three instances in the prenatal treatment of an affected fetus (21,24,45). These include the present case, a fetus with cobalamin-responsive methylmalonic acidemia (45), and another with biotin-responsive multiple carboxylase deficiency (24). It is indeed fortunate that the development of such strategies has begun with the administration of water-soluble vitamins. Complications from the use of high doses of such compounds are relatively infrequent. Known deleterious effects include: cardiovascular effects of nicotinic acid (47), oxalolithiasis with ascorbic acid (48), hypersensitivity to thiamine (49), and possible inhibition of adenosylcobalamin synthesis (50) and induction of antitranscobalamin II antibody (51) by hydroxocobalamin. Adverse effects of biotin have not been reported in humans (21). While one may therefore be optimistic in anticipating few adverse effects, caution must still be exercised, as the consequences of longer-term usage have not been completely delineated.

PRECURSOR RESTRICTION

By restricting the dietary precursors of substrates accumulating proximal to an obstruction in a metabolic pathway, it is possible to ameliorate and even prevent toxicity in a number of inborn errors of metabolism. The success of such therapy is the basis for the widespread establishment of newborn screening programs for disorders such as galactosemia and phenylketonuria (46). These two diseases will be discussed as prototypes, illustrating our capabilities and limitations in such nutritional intervention.

Galactosemia

Galactosemia is an autosomal recessive disorder of carbohydrate metabolism in which deficient galactose-1-phosphate uridyl transferase fails to convert galactose-1-phosphate to glucose-1-phosphate. There is evidence that excessively accumulating galactose-1-phosphate is the mediator of toxicity in a number of tissues (52).

A newborn with classical galactosemia does not thrive and exhibits jaundice, hepatomegaly, renal tubular dysfunction, cataracts, hemolytic anemia, seizures, and neurologic deterioration progressing to coma and death. These clinical manifestations can be remedied by withdrawing galactose from the diet before irreversible neurological deterioration occurs. Soybean-based formulas (without lactose) or other formulas containing sucrose or glucose as the carbohydrate source can be used for this purpose (53).

Treatment must be maintained throughout the lifetime of the individual. Presymptomatic dietary treatment prevents liver and kidney disease and cataracts, but may not prevent some visual defects, speech and language difficulties, EEG abnormalities, or ovarian damage (54–58). Such residual disease manifestations in well-treated individuals may be related to prenatal toxicity or to unknown deficiencies in our treatment protocols (52).

Phenylketonuria

Classical phenylketonuria (PKU) is an autosomal recessive disorder of amino acid metabolism occurring in about 1/12,000 live births (3). Deficiency of phenylalanine hydroxylase prevents synthesis of tyrosine from phenylalanine. Phenylalanine derived from dietary protein and tissue protein breakdown accumulates in physiologic fluids; it or its derivatives (e.g., phenylketones) are toxic to the nervous system (59).

During the first months of life there is little symptomatology in PKU other than a skin rash or "dry skin," and pigmentation lighter than that of the family. Between three and six months, development is noticeably delayed, with neurologic defects clearly evident by the age of one year. Microcephaly, EEG abnormalities, and frank seizures may be observed. From retrospective analyses, it is apparent that babies with phenylketonuria lose approximately 40–50 IQ points during the first year of life (60). As tyrosine cannot be synthesized, it becomes an essential amino acid. However, it is clear that phenylketonuria cannot be treated by tyrosine supplementation (61) *per se.*

Patients with untreated classical PKU evince serum phenylalanine levels over 16 mg/dl. It has been ascertained (62–64) that maintenance of blood levels between 4 and 10 mg/dl will achieve clinically satisfactory results. The desired blood phenylalanine levels can be achieved with a diet that excludes or markedly reduces sources of protein such as meat, fish, wheat, and dairy products, and which is supplemented by a protein-containing formula with a low phenylalanine content (e.g., Lofenelac®).

If the diet is initiated after the patient reaches 3 years of age, there is only behavior amelioration and little neurological or developmental improvement (64). In contrast, patients who begin dietary therapy during the first week of life, and remain on the diet at least through their first 6 years of life, perform at normal levels on school achievement tests at that time (65). In general, the effectiveness of phenylalanine restriction in classical PKU has been demonstrated in numerous studies revealing significant IQ and developmental differences between cohorts of early- and late-treated patients (60,64). However, the age at which dietary therapy for PKU can be safely discontinued has not been conclusively determined (65). Accordingly, we recommend the continuation of therapy until adolescence, at which time our uncertainties in this area can be explained to the patient.

In the extensive reports of the Los Angeles Children's Hospital Collaborative Study, the mean IQ of treated children with PKU was slightly but significantly lower than that of their unaffected siblings (62). Further, the mean IQ in the combined patient sample was slightly lower than the normative mean of 100 (63). The data suggested a small degree of relative intellectual impairment, even when treatment begins early and is properly maintained. Explanations for such residual deficits have focused on unknown defects in dietary therapy; on our incomplete understanding of the pathophysiology of the disease; and on possible prenatal damage, which we are not addressing with postnatal presymptomatic intervention. It is important to realize that even in this best characterized of inborn errors of metabolism (64), the treatment is not perfect.

Maternal Phenylketonuria

Women who have been treated for PKU during childhood are now reaching childbearing age. Such women have generally discontinued diet restrictions and are asymptomatic, with serum phenylalanine levels which may be above 20 mg/dl. Unfortunately, such high serum phenylalanine levels during pregnancy have been associated with an increased rate of spontaneous abortions and stillbirths, and with the birth of babies (heterozygotes) with low birth weight, congenital malformations, microcephaly, and developmental and mental retardation (66).

Pregnant women with PKU have been placed on phenylalanine restriction in an effort to protect the fetus against the teratogenic effects of high phenylalanine levels. Since hyperphenylalaninemic mothers with a serum phenylalanine level between 4 and 8 mg/dl show a lower incidence of significant deformities in their offspring (66,67), it was hypothesized that pregnant women with PKU should be treated so as to maintain blood phenylalanine levels in this possibly safe range. The results indicate that such dietary therapy may not be entirely protective (66,68,69). It does appear, however, that phenylalanine restriction is more effective when the diet is initiated before conception (66,68,69).

PRODUCT REPLACEMENT

When toxicity in an inborn error of metabolism results from deficiency of a product, rather than from an accumulation of a substrate, replacement therapy can be considered. Examples of such strategy include malignant hyperphenylalaninemia and Von Gierke's disease.

Malignant Hyperphenylalaninemia

Malignant hyperphenylalaninemia can be a result of defective synthesis of a cofactor (tetrahydrobiopterin) for the phenylalanine hydroxylase reaction (70), or of defective regeneration of this same cofactor because of deficient activity of dihydropteridine reductase (71). Tetrahydrobiopterin is not only a cofactor for the phenylalanine hydroxylase reaction, but is also essential for the hydroxylation of tyrosine to 3,4-dihydroxyphenylalanine (tyrosine hydroxylase), and for the hydroxylation of tryptophan to 5-hydroxytryptophan (tryptophan hydroxylase). Thus, a deficiency in available tetrahydrobiopterin may lead to defective synthesis of neurotransmitters such as dopamine, norepinephrine, and serotonin (72–75). In such patients, neurologic abnormalities are not responsive to phenylalanine restriction alone, and deterioration occurs in spite of control of serum phenylalanine levels.

Potential therapeutic approaches for malignant hyperphenylalaninemia include neurotransmitter replacement (73,74,76) and the administration of tetrahydrobiopterin (75,77), in addition to appropriate phenylalanine restriction. Clinical or chemical improvements are being reported in response to these two forms of replacement therapy in patients ascertained *after* the onset of symptoms. It is to be anticipated that truly *prospective* evaluation of such therapies will become possible as diagnoses are made earlier and presymptomatically under the auspices of newborn screening programs.

Von Gierke's Disease

A second example of product replacement strategy is the treatment of glucose-6-phosphatase deficiency (Von Gierke's disease—glycogen storage disease type IA). The glucose-6-phosphatase reaction step serves as the terminal reaction in gluconeogenesis, and as a major terminal step in the release of glucose derived from glycogenolysis. An affected child is absolutely dependent on exogenous glucose for maintenance of euglycemia (normal blood sugar) (53). The disease is characterized by hypoglycemia of variable severity, and elevations in serum uric acid, cholesterol, triglycerides, and lactate. Clinical manifestations may include hepatomegaly, growth failure, adiposity, a hemorrhagic tendency, xanthomata, and the neurologic consequences of hypoglycemia and acidosis (53).

Because many of the complications of this disorder are directly or indirectly attributable to the stimulus of hypoglycemia (78,79), therapeutic efforts have generally focused on provision of needed glucose between meals and during the nighttime hours. In a major innovation over regimens of frequent feeding or snacks, provision of glucose has most recently been accomplished by protocols utilizing continuous nocturnal intragastric infusion (79—81). The results to date have been quite promising, albeit variable, with marked improvement in blood chemistries and linear growth (79—82).

CONCLUDING REMARKS

We have reviewed capabilities and limitations of nutritional treatment approaches in inborn errors of metabolism and have commented on the timing of their application. In most inborn errors amenable to nutritional manipulation, the empiric data base is not nearly as extensive as in the disorders herein presented as examples. Nutritional restrictions, in particular, may well be deleterious in ways that are not completely understood. Therefore, in the counseling of families and discussions of prognosis, optimism may be firmly communicated but must be appropriately tempered with an honest assessment of the uncertainties that exist in such therapeutic endeavors.

In instances where vitamins have been used, we wish to emphasize that the vitamins are administered as pharmacologic agents—drugs—to treat specifically responsive inherited metabolic disorders. Even in those disorders in which the precise biochemical defect may not have been elucidated, cofactor administration is based on reasonable and focused hypotheses concerning underlying etiologies (2,4,5). Such administration is in sharp contrast to the use of "megavitamin" supplements in a random fashion in entities for which a response has not been documented, or in patients with ill-defined dysfunctions presenting no clinically valid justifications for therapeutic trials. Indiscriminate use of vitamins in pharmacologic doses—as "megavitamin" supplements—is noted here in order to firmly decry such practice as an invalid approach to patient care.

It is apparent from the foregoing that the goals of the human biochemical geneticist and nutritionist are directed not only towards the improvement and expansion of methodologies in the therapeutic repertory, but also towards the application of same at earlier and more influential stages in the ontogeny of the patient. If we consider that presymptomatic therapeutic intervention is an accepted and integral component of the management of inherited metabolic disease (46), then we can view prenatal therapy in general, and prenatal nutritional intervention in particular, as logical and reasonable extensions of such an approach to patient care. We expect that there will be an increasing number of reports of prenatal therapy of genetic disease as the precision of prenatal diagnosis continues to improve, and as more attention is given to this unique kind of opportunity to prevent disease manifestations in children.

ACKNOWLEDGMENTS

We should like to note our deep appreciation to Mr. Ardell Wallen, Mr. L. Friedman, and Ms. Beverly Cubbage for their editorial assistance and help in manuscript preparation. Certain of the work herein was supported by USPHS NIH Grant AM25884, and a grant from the March of Dimes Birth Defects Foundation.

REFERENCES

1. K. Benirschke, G. Carpenter, C. Epstein, C. Fraser, L. Jackson, A. Motulsky, and W. Nyhan, Genetic disease. In R. L. Brent and M. I. Harris, eds., *Prevention of Embryonic, Fetal, and Perinatal Disease.* DHEW Publication No. 76–853, Washington, D.C., 1976.

2. L. E. Rosenberg, Diagnosis and management of inherited aminoacidopathies in the newborn and the unborn. *Clin. Endocrinol. Metabol.* 3, 145 (1974).

3. J. B. Stanbury, J. B. Wyngaarden, D. S. Frederickson, J. L. Goldstein, and M. S. Brown, Inborn errors of metabolism in the 1980's. In J. B. Stanbury, J. B. Wyngaarden, D. S. Frederickson, J. L. Goldstein, and M. S. Brown, eds., *The Metabolic Basis of Inherited Disease,* 5th ed., McGraw-Hill, New York, 1983.

4. D. M. Danks, Management of newborn babies in whom serious metabolic illness is anticipated. *Arch. Dis. Childhood* **49**, 576 (1974).

5. Y. E. Hsia, Treatment in genetic disease. In A. Milunsky, ed., *Prevention of Genetic Disease and Mental Retardation*, W. B. Saunders, Philadelphia, 1975.

6. American Academy of Pediatrics Committee on Nutrition. *Pediatrics* **57**, 783 (1976).

7. A. E. Garrod, Inborn errors of metabolism (Croonian lectures). *Lancet* **2**, 1, 73, 142, 214 (1908).

8. M. L. Batshaw, S. Brusilow, L. Waber, W. Blom, A. M. Brubakk, B. K. Burton, H. M. Cann, D. Kerr, P. Mamunes, R. Matalon, D. Myerberg, and I. A. Schafer, Treatment of inborn errors of urea synthesis: Activation of alternative pathways of waste nitrogen synthesis and excretion. *New Engl. J. Med.* **306**, 1387–1392 (1982).

9. L. E. Rosenberg, Vitamin-responsive inherited metabolic disorders. *Adv. Human Genetics* **6**, 1 (1976).

10. L. E. Rosenberg, A. C. Lilljeqvist, and Y. E. Hsia, Methylmalonic aciduria: an inborn error leading to metabolic acidosis, long-chain ketonuria, and intermittent hyperglycinemia. *New Engl. J. Med.* **278**, 1319 (1968).

11. L. E. Rosenberg, Disorders of propionate and methylmalonate metabolism. In J. Stanbury, J. Wyngaarden, D. Frederickson, J. Goldstein, and M. Brown, eds., *The Metabolic Basis of Inherited Disease*, McGraw-Hill, New York, 1983.

12. F. X. Coude, L. Sweetman, W. Nyhan, Inhibition by propionyl CoA of N-acetylglutamate synthetase in rat liver mitochondria: A possible explanation for hyperammonemia in propionic and methylmalonic acidemia. *J. Clin. Invest.* **64**, 1544–1551 (1979).

13. S. H. Mudd, J. D. Finkelstein, F. Irrevere, and L. Laster, Homocystinuria: An enzymatic defect. *Science* **143**, 1443–1445 (1964).

14. V. A. McKusick, J. G. Hall, and F. Char, The clinical and genetic characteristics of homocystinuria. In N. Carson and D. Raine, eds., *Inherited Disorders of Sulphur Metabolism*, Edinburgh, Churchill Livingstone, 1971.

15. M. R. Seashore, J. L. Durant, and L. E. Rosenberg, Studies of the mechanism of pyridoxine-responsive homocystinuria. *Pediat. Res.* **6**, 187–196 (1972).

16. M. H. Lipson, J. Kraus, and L. E. Rosenberg, Affinity of cystathionine-β-synthetase for pyridoxal 5′-phosphate in cultured cells, a mechanism for pyridoxine-responsive homocystinuria. *J. Clin. Invest.* **66**, 188–193 (1980).

17. D. Koskow, S. Huang, and M. Lane, Propionyl holocarboxylase synthesis. *J. Biol. Chem.* **237**, 3633 (1962).

18. L. Siegel, J. Foote, and M. Coon, The enzymatic synthesis of propionyl CoA holocarboxylase from d-biotinyl 5′-adenylate and the apocarboxylase. *J. Biol. Chem.* **240**, 1025 (1965).

19. B.J. Burri, L. Sweetman, and W. Nyhan, Mutant holocarboxylase synthetase: Evidence for the enzyme defect in early infantile biotin-responsive multiple carboxylase deficiency. *J. Clin. Invest.* **68**, 1491 (1981).

20. M.E. Saunders, W.G. Sherwood, M. Duthie, L. Surh, and R.A. Gravel, Evidence for a defect of holocarboxylase synthetase activity in cultured lymphoblasts from a patient with biotin-responsive multiple carboxylase deficiency. *Am. J. Hum. Genet.* **34**, 590 (1982).

21. S. Packman, M.S. Golbus, M.J. Cowan, N.M. Caswell, L. Sweetman, B.J. Burri, W.L. Nyhan, and H. Baker, Prenatal treatment of biotin-responsive multiple carboxylase deficiency. *Lancet* **1**, 1435 (1982).

22. S. Packman, L. Sweetman, H. Baker, and S. Wall, The neonatal form of biotin-responsive multiple carboxylase deficiency. *J. Pediatr.* **99**, 418 (1981).

23. K. Roth, R. Cohn, J. Yandrasitz, F. Preti, P. Dodd, and S. Segal, Beta-methylcrotonic aciduria associated with lactic acidosis. *J. Pediatr.* **88**, 229 (1976).

24. K. Roth, W. Yang, J. Foreman, R. Rothman, and S. Segal, Holocarboxylase synthetase deficiency: A biotin-responsive organic aciduria. *J. Pediatr.* **96**, 845 (1980).

25. D. Gompertz, G.H. Draffan, J.L. Watts, and D. Hull, Biotin-responsive beta-methylcrotonylglycinuria. *Lancet* **2**, 22 (1971).

26. K. Bartlett, H. Ng, and J.V. Leonard, A combined defect of three mitrochondrial carboxylases presented as biotin-responsive 3-methylcrotonyl glycinuria and 3-hydroxyisovaleric aciduria. *Clin. Chim. Acta* **100**, 183 (1980).

27. B. Wolf, Y.E. Hsia, L. Sweetman, G. Feldman, R.B. Boychuk, R.D. Bart, D.H. Crowell, R.M. DiMauro, and W.L. Nyhan, Multiple carboxylase deficiency: Clinical and biochemical improvement following neonatal biotin treatment. *Pediatrics* **68**, 113 (1981).

28. W.G. Sherwood, M. Saunders, B.H. Robinson, T. Brewster, and R.A. Gravel, Lactic acidosis in biotin-responsive multiple carboxylase deficiency of early and late onset. *J. Pediatr.* **99**, 421 (1981).

29. S. Packman, N. Caswell, M.C. Gonzalez Rios, T. Kadlecek, H. Cann, D. Rassin, and C. McKay, Acetyl CoA carboxylase in cultured fibroblasts: Differential biotin dependence in the two types of biotin-responsive multiple carboxylase deficiency. *Am. J. Hum. Genet.* **36**, 80 (1984).

30. M. Saunder, L. Sweetman, B. Robinson, K. Roth, R. Cohn, and R. Gravel, Biotin-responsive organic aciduria: Multiple carboxylase defects and complementation studies with propionic aciduria in cultured fibroblasts. *J. Clin. Invest.* **64**, 1695 (1979).

31. S. Packman, N.M. Caswell, and H. Baker, Biochemical evidence for diverse etiologies in biotin-responsive multiple carboxylase deficiency. *Biochem. Genet.* **20**, 17 (1982).

32. W. Weyler, L. Sweetman, D. Maggio, and W. Nyhan, Deficiency of propionyl CoA carboxylase and methylcrotonyl CoA carboxylase in a

patient with methylcrotonyl glycinuria. *Clin. Chim. Acta* **76**, 321 (1971).

33. K. Bartlett and D. Gompertz, Combined carboxylase defect: Biotin-responsiveness in cultured fibroblasts. *Lancet* **2**, 804 (1976).

34. K. Bartlett and D. Gompertz, Biotin activation of carboxylase activity in cultured fibroblasts from a child with a combined carboxylase defect. *Clin. Chim. Acta* **84**, 399 (1978).

35. G. Naylor, L. Sweetman, W. Nyhan, C. Hornbeck, J. Griffiths, L. Morch, and S. Brandavage, Isotope dilution analysis of methylcitric acid in amniotic fluid for the prenatal diagnosis of propionic and methylmalonic acidemia. *Clin. Chim. Acta* **107**, 175 (1980).

36. D. W. Smith, *Recognizable Patterns of Human Malformation,* W. B. Saunders, Philadelphia, 1976.

37. H. Baker, O. Frank, A. D. Thomason, A. Langer, E. D. Munzies, B. DiAngelis, and H. A. Kaminetzky, Vitamin profile of 174 mothers and newborns at parturition. *Am. J. Clin. Nutr.* **28**, 56 (1975).

38. J. E. Sander, N. Malamud, M. J. Cowan, S. Packman, A. J. Amman, and D. W. Wara, Intermittent ataxia and immunodeficiency with multiple carboxylase deficiencies: A biotin-responsive disorder. *Ann. Neuro.* **8**, 544 (1980).

39. S. Packman, L. Sweetman, M. Yoshino, H. Baker, and M. Cowan, Biotin-responsive multiple carboxylase deficiency of infantile onset. *J. Pediatr.* **99**, 421 (1981).

40. M. J. Cowan, S. Packman, D. W. Wara, A. J. Ammann, M. Yoshino, L. Sweetman, and W. Nyhan, Multiple biotin-dependent carboxylase deficiencies associated with defects in T-cell and B-cell immunity. *Lancet* **2**, 115 (1979).

41. B. M. Charles, A. Hosking, A. Green, R. Pollit, K. Bartlett, and L. S. Taitz, Biotin-responsive alopecia and developmental regression. *Lancet* **2**, 118–120 (1979).

42. J. Thoene, H. Baker, M. Yoshino, and L. Sweetman, L-biotin responsive carboxylase deficiency associated with subnormal plasma and urinary biotin. *New Engl. J. Med.* **304**, 817–820 (1981).

43. D. Mock, A. de Lorimier, W. Liebman, L. Sweetman, and H. Baker, Biotin deficiency: An unusual complication of parenteral alimentation. *New Engl. J. Med.* **304**, 820–823 (1981).

44. B. Wolf, R. E. Grier, W. D. Parker, S. I. Goodman, and F. J. Allen, Deficient biotinidase activity in late-onset multiple carboxylase deficiency. *New Engl. J. Med.* **308**, 161 (1983).

45. M. G. Ampola, M. J. Mahoney, E. Nakamura, and K. Tanaka, Prenatal therapy of a patient with vitamin-B_{12}-responsive methylmalonic acidemia. *New Engl. J. Med.* **293**, 313 (1975).

46. H. Bickel, R. Guthrie, and G. Hammersen, eds., *Neonatal Screening for Inborn Errors of Metabolism,* Springer-Verlag, New York, 1980.

47. L. R. Mosher, Nicotinic acid side effects of toxicity, *Am. J. Psychiat.* **126**, 1290–1296 (1970).

48. M. Lamden and G. Chrystowski, Urinary oxalate excretion by man following ascorbic acid ingestion, *Proc. Soc. Exp. Biol. Med.* **85**, 1190–1192 (1954).

49. A.G. Gilman, L.S. Goodman, and A. Gilman, eds., *The Pharmacological Basis of Therapeutics*, Macmillan, New York, 1980.

50. M.J. Mahoney, J.F. Nicholson, J.C. Hart, L.E. Rosenberg, and R. Challop. Cobalamin (vitamin B_{12}) toxicity in methylmalonicacidemia. *Pediatr. Res.* **10**, 368 (1976).

51. A.P. Skouby, E. Hippe, and H. Olesen. Antibody to transcobalamin II and B_{12} binding capacity in patients treated with hydroxocobalamin. *Blood* **38**, 769–774 (1971).

52. G.M. Komrower, Galactosaemia—Thirty years or the experience of a generation. *J. Inher. Metab. Dis.* suppl. **2**, 96–104 (1982).

53. M. Cornblath and R. Schwartz, *Disorders of Carbohydrate Metabolism in Infancy*, W.B. Saunders, Philadelphia, 1976.

54. K. Fishler, R. Kock, G.N. Donnell, and E. Wenz, Developmental aspects of galactosemia from infancy to childhood. *Clin. Pediatr.* **19**, 38 (1980).

55. S. Waisbren, T. Norman, R. Schnell, and H. Levy, Speech and language deficits in early-treated children with galactosemia. *J. Pediatr.* **102**, 75 (1983).

56. F.R. Kaufman, M.D. Kogut, G.N. Donnell, U. Goebelsmann, C. March, and R. Koch, Hypergonadotropic hypogonadism in female patients with galactosemia. *New Engl. J. Med.* **304**, 994 (1981).

57. Y.T. Chen, D.R. Mattison, and J.D. Schulman, Hypogonadism and galactosemia. *New Engl. J. Med.* **305**, 464 (1981).

58. B. Steinmann, R. Gitzelmann, and M. Zachmann, Hypogonadism and galactosemia, *New Engl. J. Med.* **305**, 464 (1981).

59. F.A. Hommes, A.G. Eller, and E.H. Taylor, Turnover of the fast components of myelin and myelin products in experimental hyperphenylalanemia. Relevance to termination of dietary treatment in human phenylketonuria. *J. Inher. Metab. Dis.* **5**, 21 (1982).

60. C.R. Scriver and L.E. Rosenberg, *Amino Acid Metabolism and Its Disorders*, W.B. Saunders, Philadelphia, 1973.

61. M.L. Batshaw, D. Valle, and S.P. Bessman, Unsuccessful treatment of phenylketonuria with tyrosine. *J. Pediatrics* **99**, 159–160 (1981).

62. J.C. Dobson, E. Kushida, M. Williamson, and E. Friedman, Intellectual performance of 36 phenylketonuria patients and their parents and their nonaffected siblings. *Pediatrics* **58**, 53 (1976).

63. J.C. Dobson, M.L. Williamson, C. Azen, and R. Koch, Intellectual assessment of 111 four year old children with phenylketonuria. *Pediatrics* **60**, 822 (1977).

64. C.R. Scriver and C.L. Clow, Phenylketonuria: The epitome of human biochemical genetics. *New Engl. J. Med.* **303**, 1336 and 1394 (1980).

65. R. Koch, C.G. Azen, E.G. Friedman, and M.L. Williamson, Preliminary report on the effects of diet discontinuation in PKU. *J. Pediatr.* **100**, 870 (1982).

66. R. R. Lenke and H. L. Levy, Maternal phenylketonuria and hyperphenylalaninemia: An international survey of the outcome of untreated and treated pregnancies. *New Engl. J. Med.* **303**, 1202 (1980).

67. P. B. Acosta, M. Blaskovics, H. Cloud, E. Lis, H. Stroud, and E. Wenz, Nutrition in pregnancy of women with hyperphenylalaninemia. *J. Am. Diet. Assoc.* **80**, 443 (1982).

68. H. L. Levy, G. N. Kaplan, and A. M. Erickson, Comparison of treated and untreated pregnancies in mothers with PKU. *J. Pediatr.* **100**, 876 (1982).

69. R. Lenke and H. Levy, Maternal phenylketonuria—Results of dietary therapy. *Am. J. Obstet. Gynec.* **142**, 548 (1982).

70. S. Kaufman, S. Berlow, G. K. Summer, S. Milstien, J. D. Schulman, S. Orloff, S. Spielberg, and S. Pueschel, Hyperphenylalaninemia due to a deficiency of biopterin: A variant form of phenylketonuria. *New Engl. J. Med.* **299**, 673 (1978).

71. S. Kaufman, N. A. Holtzman, S. Milstien, I. J. Butler, and A. Krumholz, Phenylketonuria due to a deficiency of dihydropteridine reductase. *New Engl. J. Med.* **293**, 785 (1975).

72. S. H. Koslow and I. J. Butler, Biogenic amine synthesis defect in dihydropteridine reductase deficiency. *Science* **198**, 522—523 (1977).

73. I. J. Butler, S. H. Koslow, A. Krumholz, N. A. Holtzman, and S. Kaufman, A disorder of biogenic amines in dihydropteridine reductase deficiency. *Ann. Neurol.* **3**, 224÷230 (1978).

74. T. Tanaka, K. Aihana, K. Iwai, M. Kohashi, K. Tomita, K. Narisawa, N. Arai, H. Yoshida, and T. Uui, Hyperphenylalaninemia due to impaired dihydrobiopterin biosynthesis. *Eur. J. Ped.* **136**, 275—280 (1981).

75. D. M. Danks, P. Schlesinger, F. Firgaira, R. G. H. Cotton, B. M. Watson, H. Rembold, and G. Hennings, Malignant hyperphenylalaninemia—Clinical features, biochemical findings, and experience with administration of biopterins. *Pediatr. Res.* **13**, 1150—1155 (1979).

76. K. Bartholomé, D. J. Byrd, S. Kaufman, and S. Milstien, Atypical phenylketonuria with normal phenylalanine hydroxylase and dihydropteridine reductase activity *in vitro*. *Pediatrics* **59**, 757—761 (1977).

77. S. Kaufman, G. Kapatos, R. McInnes, J. D. Schulman, and W. Rizzo, Use of tetrahydropterins in the treatment of hyperphenylalaninemia due to defective synthesis of tetrahydrobiopterin: Evidence that peripherally administered tetrahydropterins enter the brain. *Pediatrics* **70**, 376—380 (1982).

78. P. Blackett, Secondary metabolic changes in Von Gierke's disease. *Ann. Clin. Lab. Science* **12**, 424—430 (1982).

79. H. L. Greene, A. E. Slonim, J. A. O'Neill, Jr., and I. M. Burr, Continuous nocturnal intragastric feeding for management of type 1 glycogen-storage disease. *New Engl. J. Med.* **294**, 423—425 (1976).

80. H. L. Greene, A. E. Slonim, I. M. Burr, and J. R. Moran, Type I glycogen storage disease: Five years of management with nocturnal intragastric feeding. *J. Pediatr.* **96**, 590—595 (1980).

81. J. F. Crigler, Jr. and J. Folkman, Glycogen storage disease: New approaches to therapy. *Ciba Foundation Symposium, No. 55*, 331–356, (1977).

82. V. V. Michels, A. L. Beaudet, V. E. Potts, and C. M. Montandon, Glycogen storage disease: Long-term follow-up of nocturnal intragastric feeding. *Clin. Genet.* **21**, 136–140 (1982).

5

Variation in Serum Cholesterol Levels

DAVID KRITCHEVSKY, Ph.D.

The Wistar Institute of Anatomy and Biology
Philadelphia, Pennsylvania

Address correspondence to David Kritchevsky, Ph.D., The Wistar Institute of Anatomy and Biology, 36th Street at Spruce, Philadelphia, Pennsylvania 19104.

ABSTRACT

One of the major risk factors for coronary heart disease is an elevated plasma cholesterol level. As early as 1924 it was observed that cholesterol levels fluctuated with an apparent seasonal rhythm. Since 1924 many investigators have studied this phenomenon. Most of the investigations find fluctuations in serum cholesterol levels. Seasonal variations are often seen but the reported variations do not occur at the same time of year in all experiments. Cholesterol levels may vary by 30% or more, although the usual swings are closer to $\pm 15\%$. The intra-individual variations are reflected in the levels of high-density lipoprotein cholesterol as well as in total cholesterol. The reason(s) for the swings are unclear but stress seems to play an important role. The data suggest that a single determination of serum or plasma cholesterol is not sufficient basis for diagnosis of coronary disease or assessment of treatment.

There is a story of a would-be bank robber who presented the teller with a note which read, "This is a stick-up. Hand me your money. Act normal." The teller returned the note with the comment, "Define normal." The question of what value for blood parameters is normal or is in the normal range continues to pique investigators. A case in point is the variation of serum or plasma cholesterol levels, which fluctuate just often enough to keep us wary.

One of the undisputed major risk factors for coronary heart disease is elevated serum or plasma cholesterol level (1). A major medical effort is directed towards reduction of cholesterol levels in hopes of ameliorating the course of coronary heart disease. The purpose of this essay is not to question this firmly established hypothesis, but rather to review again the data pertinent to the establishment of basal or normal

---

Research supported, in part, by a Research Career Award (HL-00734) from the National Institutes of Health and by funds from the Commonwealth of Pennsylvania.

cholesterol levels. This important subject is addressed every few years. Cholesterol levels tend to vary—diurnally, seasonally, and under stress—so that a determination at only one point in time may be misleading. Even more bothersome is the fact that the variation appears to be random, so that there is no predictable formula one can apply.

In 1924, Currie (2) studied cholesterol levels in cancer patients and controls and found a seasonal rhythm in both groups. Levels observed between November and January were 39% lower than those seen between February and April. Cholesterol levels of the cancer patients were lower (17–30%) than those of the normal controls at every time period. In 1936 Schube (3) studied cholesterol levels in 10 men for a period of 16 weeks. While the average for the group was remarkably constant, individual levels tended to vary by as much as 31%. Only

Table 1. Individual Cholesterol Values in Young Prisoners (Measured monthly over one year)[a]

Subject Number[b]	Mean Serum Cholesterol (mg/dl ± SD)	Range
1	179 ± 15	148–205
2	182 ± 18	148–212
3	191 ± 29	170–278
4	200 ± 16	175–225
5	211 ± 20	175–240
6	218 ± 19	180–248
7	218 ± 25	170–255
8	219 ± 25	180–270
9	233 ± 25	200–270
10	234 ± 22	205–278
11	247 ± 25	225–315
12	261 ± 27	225–315
13	296 ± 50	225–375
14	300 ± 41	233–375
15	301 ± 38	248–387
16	308 ± 37	255–365

[a] After Thomas et al. (9).
[b] Subjects 1-8—low cholesterol group (<225 mg/dl).
Subjects 9-12—intermediate cholesterol group (225–274 mg/dl).
Subjects 13-16—high cholesterol group (>275 mg/dl).

Table 2. Seasonal Variation of Serum Cholesterol[a]

Month	Mean Serum Cholesterol[b] (mg/dl ± SD)	Coefficient of Variation (%)
April	227 ± 51	22.4
May	217 ± 48	21.9
June	215 ± 46	21.5
July	211 ± 49	23.2
August	226 ± 51	22.6
September	227 ± 47	20.8
October	232 ± 51	22.2
November	233 ± 54	23.2
December	224 ± 50	22.2
January	226 ± 52	22.8
February	233 ± 53	22.7
March	225 ± 50	22.0

[a] After Doyle et al. (10).
[b] Fifty two subjects.

three subjects showed maximum variations of less than 20%. Sperry (4) found variations of up to 28% in a group of men he studied. Thompson et al. (5) studied a small number of normal subjects and patients with coronary disease (10 and 14 subjects, respectively) and found deviations from the mean of over 25%. They suggested that at least four or five determinations of serum cholesterol should be performed in order to establish a baseline level. Extent of variation did not appear to be influenced by coronary heart disease (5,6).

In 1958, Levere et al. (7) reported a study of plant sterol effects on hypercholesterolemia. They described such wide fluctuations in cholesterol levels that it made interpretation of their results hazardous. Consequently, they were unable to ascribe any decrease in cholesterol level to medication. They studied 25 patients for a period of 9–23 months (average 15.5) and found swings in cholesterol levels of 21.4% above (range 10–39) and 19.6% below (range 11–33) the median cholesterol level of 247 ± 8 mg/dl.

Paloheimo (8) described seasonal variation of serum cholesterol in a group of 44 Finnish policemen. Cholesterol levels were elevated from January through March and then fell to a low level in May. Cholesterol levels rose again in September, reaching a peak in October and November. Thomas et al. (9) studied the cholesterol levels of 16 convicts in Maryland and found a variation in cholesterol levels similar to that seen by Paloheimo (8). Cholesterol levels were elevated in the

Table 3. Seasonal Variation of Serum Cholesterol Levels [a]

Month	Serum Cholesterol (mg/dl)	
	1965	1966
January	250	269
February	257	264
March	268	260
April	251	269
May	241	269
June	236	263
July	246	269
August	233	245
September	225	239
October	236	233
November	242	237
December	259	235

[a] After Fyfe et al. (11).
(Values extrapolated from graph.)

Table 4. Seasonal Variation in Serum Lipids [a]

Month	Lipids (mg/dl) [b]	
	Cholesterol	Triglyceride
January	207	98
February	192	100
March	200	85
April	201	89
May	200	72
June	203	73
July	204	79
August	195	87
September	194	90
October	189	90
November	206	73
December	209	71

[a] After Warnick and Albers (14).
[b] Mean of two analyses: Eleven subjects.
(Values extrapolated from graph).

winter months and low in the summer. They found a resemblance between a graph of monthly cholesterol levels and patterns of deaths from coronary disease in the United States. Their data are summarized in Table 1. Doyle et al. (10) assayed serum total cholesterol in 52 healthy middle-aged males. Their results (Table 2) show the lowest average level in July (211 ±54.3 mg/dl) and the highest in November (233 ±54.3 mg/dl) and February (233 ±52.8 mg/dl). Fyfe et al. (11) reported on a total of 3701 observations carried out over a two-year period on an unspecified number of subjects. They found the peak cholesterol level to occur in March and April and the trough in September and October (Table 3). Carlson and Lindstedt (12) measured cholesterol levels in over 2000 Swedish men and women and found peak levels to occur in October and November and the lowest levels to occur in July. The patterns of variation with season were similar in men and women.

Green et al. (13) reported on cholesterol levels in subjects observed over a nine-month period. Readings (894 in all) were obtained as the subjects entered a clinical trial of a hypolipidemic drug (Atromid). Peak cholesterol levels (360 mg/dl) were observed in August and the lowest levels (300 mg/dl) in March.

Warnick and Albers (14) studied the plasma cholesterol and triglyceride levels of 11 healthy subjects over a one-year period. Analytical variation was small, 1–2% for cholesterol and 2–5% for triglycerides. A significant ($p < 0.05$) seasonal trend was observed, with cholesterol being highest in the winter months and lowest in October (Table 4). They conceded that "...intra-individual variation can be an important source of error in attempting to make a genetic diagnosis of hyperlipidemia and/or in evaluating hypolipidemic regimens in a given subject."

The variations in cholesterol levels are reflected in changes in lipoprotein and apolipoprotein levels as well. Van Gent et al. (15) studied seasonal variation in high-density lipoprotein cholesterol (HDL-C) levels in forty-year-old citizens of Leiden; there were 533 men and 494 women in the study. The curves for men and women were qualitatively similar. In men, the mean HDL-C level was 42.5 ±10.7 mg/dl, and in women it was 48.0 ±11.0 mg/dl. Significantly lower levels were observed in March for both sexes. HDL-C levels were significantly higher than the mean in June (women) and July (men). Fager et al. (16) determined serum total cholesterol, HDL-C, and apolipoproteins A-I, A-II, and B in 12 men. Total serum cholesterol and HDL-C were lower in the winter (December). The apolipoprotein levels, on the other hand, were lower in the summer months and higher in the winter.

Harlap and his colleagues (17) have reported on seasonal variations in plasma lipid and lipoprotein levels in 5246 subjects being studied in the Jerusalem Lipid Research Clinic. In men (2459), peak levels of total cholesterol were in October and December, with the lowest levels being observed in June. Low-density lipoprotein (LDL) cholesterol levels also peaked in October and were lowest in July. HDL-C levels were highest in January, March, and December and lowest in July. The ratio of HDL-C to total cholesterol was highest in January and lowest in October (Table 5). In the female subjects (2787), the patterns were qualitatively similar to those observed in the male group. The authors concluded: "...clinicians should take season into account when diagnosing hyperlipidemia and when evaluating success or failure in its treatment. Studies of lipid distributions and of interventions aimed at lipid modification need to consider the potentially compounding effects of season...."

Table 5. Seasonal Variation of Plasma Lipid and Lipoprotein Levels (Men)[a]

Month	Subjects	Cholesterol[b]	HDL-Cholesterol[b]
1	208	200.6	43.1
2	156	202.9	41.6
3	191	201.6	42.3
4	125	199.3	41.2
5	315	197.0	40.4
6	338	194.2	39.5
7	288	194.9	39.3
8	273	198.7	40.9
9	138	199.2	40.2
10	77	209.8	41.0
11	170	202.1	41.3
12	180	205.0	42.7

[a] After Harlap et al. (17).
[b] Adjusted for age, Quetelet index, origin group, and social class.

Seasonal variation of cholesterol levels is not a universal finding. McEachern and Gilmour (18) flatly stated, in 1932, that seasonal variations did not exist. Turner and Steiner (19) found no diurnal variation in their subjects. They determined cholesterol levels during control periods of about two months interspersed with treatment with either potassium iodide or thyroid hormone preparation. Although they comment on the relative constancy of cholesterol levels during the control periods, their data show that the reading deviated from the average by as much as −15.4 or +12.5%. Lund et al. (20) reported on a study of 637 male and 163 female subjects in Copenhagen whose

Table 6. Summary of Observed Seasonal Variations in Cholesterol Levels

Number of Cases	Time (Months)	Peak	Trough	Reference
67	12	May—July	Nov.—Jan.	2
80	12	Mar.; Nov.	May—Aug.	8
16	12	Nov.—Jan.	May—Oct.	9
637	12	July; Jan.	Dec.	20
201	9	Aug.	Dec.; Mar.	13
52	12	Nov.; Feb.	July	10
a	24	Mar.—Apr.	Sept.—Oct.	11
6464	12	Sept.—Oct.	June—July	12
1005	15	Dec.	Oct.	22
11	13	Dec.	Oct.	14
12	21	July—Aug.	Jan.; Dec.	16
5246	12	Nov.	June—July	17

a 3701 estimations.

cholesterol levels were followed from March 1959 to March 1960. They concluded no seasonal variations were observed; however, extrapolation from a graph of their findings shows that cholesterol levels of the male subjects were about 245 mg/dl in March, 1959; 205 mg/dl in June, 1959; 190 mg/dl in December, 1959; 235 mg/dl in January, 1960; and 225 mg/dl in March, 1960. Cholesterol levels in the female subjects were much less variable but ranged from 215 mg/dl in March of 1959 to 243 mg/dl in August of 1959, and 250 mg/dl in March of 1960.

Samuel et al. (21) studied cholesterol levels for one year in 12 patients with atherosclerosis. The average monthly levels were remarkably constant; however, they found significant individual variations that were totally erratic. There was no variation coinciding with change of season.

Fuller et al. (22) studied two different groups of subjects and found no differences between cholesterol levels determined in spring or autumn (group 1, 80 subjects) or in summer and winter (group 2, 73 subjects). They did find variations in triglyceride levels that could not be ascribed to changes in weight or diets. Their plot of fasting plasma cholesterol levels for their entire cohort showed a range from 230 mg/dl in October and February to 257 mg/dl in December.

Mjøs et al. (23) studied a number of lipoprotein parameters in 28 subjects over a period of 60 weeks. They found no variation in total serum cholesterol. Demacker et al. (24) found intra-individual variations of cholesterol ranging from 3.9 to 10.9% and HDL-C ranging from 3.6 to 12.4% in 53 normal subjects studied for a period of one year. They saw no significant diurnal or seasonal variations.

The foregoing suggests that there are real intra-individual variations in serum cholesterol and HDL-C levels which may or may not be seasonal in nature. Ripley (25) suggests that some of the reports may have suffered from methodological inadequacies or mathematical artifacts. However, everyone cautions against diagnosis based on single determinations. There is probably something to be said for assessment of reports based on the number of subjects, which has ranged from 10 to over 5000. Table 6 summarizes the reported seasonal variations. Seasonal variations in cholesterol level have also been observed in the rat (26), monkey (27), baboon (28), woodchuck (29), and badger (30).

Assuming the admitted intra-individual variations in serum cholesterol, the source of these variations becomes of importance. Diet does not appear to play a significant role (22,31). Reinberg et al. (32) found seasonal variations in plasma levels of a number of hormones including (peak): FSH (February), LH (March), thyroxine (September), cortisol (February), renin (April), and testosterone (October). There might be a direct or inverse relationship between plasma lipid levels and hormonal activity. Persson (33) found seasonal variations in lipoprotein lipase activity of human subcutaneous adipose tissue. Lipoprotein lipase activity was high in January and October and low in July and August.

Stressful situations have been shown to exert a hypercholesterolemic effect in otherwise normal subjects. The stress of impending examinations results in significant elevation of cholesterol levels in medical students (34,35). In their classic study of occupational stress in accountants, Friedman et al. (36) demonstrated hypercholesterolemic effects of periods of work stress. One individual showed an increase of serum cholesterol from 231 mg/dl to 326 mg/dl in a period of two weeks. Groover et al. (37) studied 177 individuals over a period of 5 years and obtained at least six cholesterol determinations per year from each subject. Cholesterol variation over that period averaged 25% with 38 of the individuals exhibiting less than 20% variation and 37 of the individuals showing more than 50% variation. There were 16 myocardial infarctions in the group and all occurred in men whose plasma cholesterol levels varied 55% or more. Myocardial infarction was correlated with maximum fluctuations (Table 7). One of the subjects exhibited cholesterol levels that fluctuated between 100 mg/dl and 800 mg/dl over the period of study (38).

Table 7. Variation of Cholesterol Level (177 subjects studied over a 5-year period) [a]

Percent Variation	Number of Subjects	Myocardial Infarction
0–9	9	0
10–19	29	0
20–29	47	0
30–39	31	0
40–49	24	0
50–59	12	1
60–69	8	3
70–79	5	2
80–89	5	4
90–99	4	3
100+	3	3
	177	16

[a]After Groover et al. (37).

What conclusions can be drawn? Principally, that individual serum cholesterol levels tend to vary, often widely. The variations may be seasonal in nature, but they occur even when rhythmic periodicity cannot be observed. The cause of the fluctuations is undefined, although stress has been implicated in a number of instances. Physiological factors may also play a role, but there are few data on this subject. However, the admonition made in several of the cited papers should be heeded, namely, a single determination is insufficient basis for diagnosis of disease or assessment of treatment. It may be possible to address this problem in animal studies by attempting to correlate the activities of the critical enzymes of cholesterol synthesis (3-hydroxy-3-methylglutaryl CoA reductase) and degradation (cholesterol 7α-hydroxylase) with variations of serum cholesterol levels.

REFERENCES

1. A. Kagan, W. B. Kannel, T. R. Dawber, and N. Revotskie, The coronary profile. *Ann. N.Y. Acad. Sci.* **97**, 883 (1962).
2. A. N. Currie, The cholesterol of blood in malignant disease. *Br. J. Exp. Path.* **5**, 293 (1924).
3. P. G. Schube, Variations in the blood cholesterol of man over a period of time. *J. Lab. Clin. Med.* **22**, 280 (1936).
4. W. M. Sperry, The concentration of total cholesterol in the blood serum. *J. Biol. Chem.* **117**, 391 (1937).

5.   J.S. Thompson, A. Abraham, A.W. Elias, and C.C. Scott, Observations on the variations of total serum cholesterol levels in normal individuals and in patients with heart disease. *Am. J. Med. Sci.* **237**, 319 (1959).

6.   J.B. Cromie, K.J. Thomson, O.S. Cullimore, and E.F. Beach, Studies in serum lipids with special reference to spontaneous variation and effect of short term dietary changes. *Circulation* **27**, 360 (1963).

7.   A.H. Levere, R.C. Boziran, G. Craft, R.S. Jackson, and C.F. Wilkinson, Jr., The "Sitosterols": Variability of serum cholesterol levels and difficulty of evaluating decholesterolizing agents. *Metabolism* **7**, 338 (1958).

8.   J. Paloheimo, Seasonal variations of serum lipids in healthy men. *Ann. Med. Exp. Fenn.* **39** (Suppl. 8), 1 (1961).

9.   C.B. Thomas, H.W.D. Holljes, and F.A. Eisenberg, Observations on seasonal variations in total serum cholesterol level among healthy young prisoners. *Ann. Intern. Med.* **54**, 413 (1961).

10. J.T. Doyle, S.H. Kinch, and D.F. Brown, Seasonal variation in serum cholesterol concentration. *J. Chronic Dis.* **18**, 657 (1965).

11. T. Fyfe, M.G. Dunnigan, E. Hamilton, and R.J. Rae, Seasonal variation in serum lipids and incidence and mortality of ischaemic heart disease. *J. Atheroscler. Res.* **8**, 591 (1968).

12. L.A. Carlson and S. Lindstedt, The Stockholm Prospective Study. 1. The initial values for plasma lipids. *Acta Med. Scand. Suppl.* **493**, 1 (1968).

13. K.G. Green, W.H.W. Inman, and J.M. Thorp, Multicentre trial in the United Kingdom and Ireland of a mixture of ethyl chlorophenoxyisobutyrate and androsterone (Atromid). A preliminary report. *J. Atheroscler. Res.* **3**, 593 (1963).

14. G.R. Warnick and J.J. Albers, Physiological and analytical variation in cholesterol and triglycerides. *Lipids* **11**, 203 (1976).

15. C.M. Van Gent, H. Van Der Voort, and L.W. Hessel, High density lipoprotein cholesterol, monthly variation and association with cardiovascular risk factors in 1000 forty-year-old Dutch citizens. *Clin. Chim. Acta* **88**, 155 (1978).

16. G. Fagar, O. Wiklund, S.O. Olofsson, and G. Bondjers, Seasonal variations in serum lipid and apolipoprotein levels evaluated by periodic regression analyses. *J. Chronic Dis.* **35**, 643 (1982).

17. S. Harlap, J.D. Kark, M. Baras, S. Eisenberg, and Y. Stein, Seasonal changes in plasma lipid and lipoprotein levels in Jerusalem. *Israel J. Med. Sci.* **18**, 1158 (1982).

18. J.M. McEachern and C.R. Gilmour, Studies in cholesterol metabolism. 2. Blood cholesterol in various conditions. *Can. Med. Assoc. J.* **26**, 158 (1932).

19. K.B. Turner and A. Steiner, A long term study of the variation of serum cholesterol in man. *J. Clin. Invest.* **18**, 45 (1939).

20. E. Lund, T. Geill, and P.H. Andresen, Serum cholesterol in normal subjects in Denmark. *Lancet* **2**, 1383 (1961).

21. P. Samuel, S. Lieberman, F.S. Shmase, E. Meilman, and G. Toufexis, Variation in total serum cholesterol concentration in patients with atherosclerosis. *Am. J. Clin. Nutr.* **23**, 178 (1970).

22. J.H. Fuller, S.L. Grainger, R.J. Jarrett, and H. Keen, Possible seasonal variation of plasma lipids in a healthy population. *Clin. Chem. Acta* **52**, 305 (1974).

23. O.D. Mjøs, S.N. Rao, L. Bjoru, T. Henden, D.S. Thelle, O.H. Forde, and N.E. Miller, A longitudinal study of the biological variability of plasma lipoproteins in healthy young adults. *Atherosclerosis* **34**, 75 (1979).

24. P.N.M. Demacker, R.W.B. Schade, R.T.P. Jansen, and A. Van't Loar, Intra-individual variation of serum cholesterol, triglycerides and high density lipoprotein cholesterol in normal humans. *Atherosclerosis* **45**, 259 (1982).

25. R.M. Ripley, Overview: Seasonal variation in cholesterol. *Preventive Med.* **10**, 665 (1981).

26. J.M. Thorp, Effects of seasonal variation on lipid metabolism in animals and man. In J.K. Grant, ed., *The Control of Lipid Metabolism*, Academic Press, London, 1963, pp. 163–168.

27. D. Kritchevsky and R.F.J. McCandless, Weekly variations in serum cholesterol levels of monkeys. *Proc. Soc. Exp. Biol. Med.* **95**, 152 (1957).

28. D. Kritchevsky, E.S. Kritchevsky, P.P. Nair, J.A. Jastremsky, and I.L. Shapiro, Effect of free fatty acids on cholesterol metabolism in the baboon. *Nutr. Dieta* **9**, 283 (1967).

29. G.M. Wenberg and J.C. Holland, The circannual variations in the total serum lipids and cholesterol with respect to body weight in the woodchuck (*Marmota Monax*). *Comp. Biochem. Physiol.* **44A**, 577 (1973).

30. P.M. Laplaud, L. Beaubatie, and D. Maurel, A spontaneously seasonal hypercholesterolemic animal: Plasma lipids and lipoproteins in the European badger (*Meles meles* L.). *J. Lipid Res.* **21**, 724 (1980).

31. M.W. Porter, W. Yamanaka, S.D. Carlson, and M.A. Flynn, Effect of dietary egg on serum cholesterol and triglyceride of human males. *Am. J. Clin.* **30**, 490 (1977).

32. A Reinberg, M. Lagoguey, F. Cesselin, Y. Touitou, J.C. Legrand, A. Delassalle, J. Antreassian, and A. Lagoguey. Circadian and circannual rhythms in plasma hormones and other variables of five healthy young human males. *Acta Endocrinologica* **88**, 417 (1978).

33. B. Persson, Seasonal variation of lipoprotein lipase activity in human subcutaneous adipose tissue. *Clin. Sci. Molec. Med.* **47**, 631 (1974).

34. C.B. Thomas and E.A. Murphy, Further studies on cholesterol levels in the Johns Hopkins medical students: The effect of stress at examinations. *J. Chronic Dis.* **8**, 661 (1958).

35. P.T. Wertlake, A.A. Wilcox, M.I. Haley, and J.E. Peterson, Relationship of mental and emotional stress to serum cholesterol levels. *Proc. Soc. Exp. Biol. Med.* **97**, 163 (1958).

36. M. Friedman, R.H. Rosenman, and V. Carroll, Changes in the serum

cholesterol and blood clotting time in men subjected to cyclic variation of occupational stress. *Circulation* **17**, 852 (1958).

37. M. E. Groover, Jr., J. A. Jernigan, and C. D. Martin, Variations in serum lipid concentration and clinical coronary disease. *Am. J. Med. Sci.* **239**, 133 (1960).

38. M. E. Groover, Jr., Clinical evaluation of a public health program to prevent coronary artery disease. *Trans. College of Physicians of Philadelphia*, Fourth Series, **24**, 105 (1956–7).

SECTION TWO
Nutrient Update

6

Ultratrace Elements
CURRENT STATUS

FORREST H. NIELSEN, Ph.D.

Research Chemist
U.S. Department of Agriculture
Agricultural Research Service
Grand Forks Human Nutrition Research Center
Grand Forks, North Dakota

Address correspondence to Forrest H. Nielsen, Ph.D., U.S. Department of Agriculture, Agricultural Research Service, Grand Forks Human Nutrition Research Center, P.O. Box 7166, University Station, Grand Forks, North Dakota 58202.

ABSTRACT

Review of the experimental evidence supporting the suggestion of nutritional essentiality of 11 ultratrace elements for both animals and humans indicates that only arsenic, nickel, and silicon meet the definition of essentiality. Some evidence suggests that boron, lithium, and vanadium are also essential nutrients. There is no sound evidence to support the nutritional essentiality of bromine, cadmium, fluorine, lead, and tin; however, certain benefits of fluorine are well known. Further research is needed to establish whether the ultratrace elements have a more important role in human health than is now generally acknowledged.

BACKGROUND

Since 1970, scientists have suggested that at least 11 elements could be added to the list of trace elements that are nutritionally essential. Estimated dietary requirements for these elements are usually less than 1 $\mu g/g$, and often are less than 50 ng/g. Those elements, which have been designated as ultratrace elements, are arsenic, boron, bromine, cadmium, fluorine, lead, lithium, nickel, silicon, tin, and vanadium. Although deficiency in humans has not been described for any of those ultratrace elements, some attention has been directed toward the possibility that some of them might be the missing links in some unexplained human diseases. The finding of a severe uncompounded deficiency of any ultratrace element that causes an acute disease seems unlikely. However, situations other than a simple acute deficiency might make these elements of nutritional significance for humans. These situations include: (1) inborn errors of metabolism that affect absorption, retention, and excretion; (2) alterations in metabolism and/or biochemistry as a secondary consequence to malnutrition, disease, injury, or stress; (3) inadvertent omission from a total parenteral nutrition solution; and (4) marginal deficiencies (slight deviation from an optimal intake of an essential nutrient) induced by various dietary manipulations or by direct or indirect interaction with another nutrient or drug. Thus, those who are concerned with human nutrition should be aware of the current status of research on ultratrace element nutrition, or the quality of the experimental evidence supporting the suggestion of nutritional essentiality, which varies widely among the ultratrace elements. In this review, an element is considered essential if a dietary deficiency of that element consistently results in a suboptimal biological function that is preventable or reversible by physiological amounts of the element.

ARSENIC

Reviews summarizing the signs of arsenic deprivation for four animal species—chick, goat, minipig, and rat—were recently published (1–3). In the goat, minipig, and rat, the most consistent signs of arsenic deprivation were depressed growth, and abnormal reproduction characterized by impaired fertility and elevated perinatal mortality. Other notable signs of deprivation in goats were depressed serum triglycerides and death during lactation. Histologic examination revealed myocardial damage in the lactating goats that died.

Studies with chicks indicated that the extent, severity, and direction of the signs of arsenic deprivation were affected by the arginine and zinc status of the animal (3). For example, the effect of dietary arsenic on growth depended upon the zinc status of the chick. Arsenic deprivation did not markedly affect growth when dietary zinc was luxuriant (>50 μg/g), but depressed growth when dietary zinc was marginally adequate (25–40 μg/g). During severe zinc deficiency, growth was more markedly depressed in arsenic-supplemented than in arsenic-deprived chicks.

No specific biological role for arsenic has been found. However, findings with chicks suggest that arsenic has a role in the metabolism of arginine and zinc. Possibly this role involves amino acid or protein metabolism. The suggestive findings include that arsenic deprivation elevated plasma uric acid in chicks fed luxuriant zinc but depressed plasma uric acid in chicks fed less than 40 μg zinc/g of diet (3). Chicks usually eliminate excess amino acid nitrogen as uric acid. Arsenic deprivation depressed total microsomal protein in the livers of chicks and rats (4), and the "raw" protein level in minipigs (5). Arsenic deprivation depressed the level of arginine and elevated the level of lysine in the plasma of chicks (E. O. Uthus, personal communication).

Although a specific biochemical function for arsenic is unknown, data from studies done in three different laboratories and on four different animal species show that arsenic is an essential nutrient for experimental animals. The possible importance of arsenic in human nutrition can only be inferred from the results of animal studies. Generally, extrapolation of experimental findings from animals to humans is difficult. For the major trace elements that are clearly required by humans, however, signs of deficiency often correspond closely with signs observed in experimental animals. Possibly, therefore, arsenic and other ultratrace elements that are essential for animals are also essential for humans. Furthermore, some of the deficiency signs and requirements described for animals might have counterparts for humans. The arsenic requirement for chicks apparently is less than 50 ng/g of diet and probably near 25 ng/g (1). Based on animal data, a possible arsenic requirement for humans would be about 12–25 μg daily.

Tabulations of the arsenic content of a number of foods show that most diets probably provide adequate amounts of arsenic if the requirements of humans are similar to those suggested for chicks. Early estimates of the oral intake of arsenic by humans (400–900 μg/day) (6) were most likely too high. Subsequent surveys, which indicate an intake of 20–130 μg/day, may be more realistic (7,8). Diets high in fish and seafood would contain much more arsenic than diets high in dairy products, certain vegetables, and fruits.

It is inappropriate to suggest specific disorders in which abnormal arsenic nutrition is a contributing factor until more is known about its physiological function. At present, it is probably most important to be aware of the likelihood that arsenic is essential for humans. Arsenic has been synonymous with poison for centuries, and recently, associated with some forms of cancer. Beliefs that any form, or amount, of arsenic is unnecessary, toxic, or carcinogenic might lead to efforts for a zero-base exposure to arsenic, or for elimination of as much arsenic as possible from dietary sources for humans. The consequence of eliminating an essential nutrient from the diet is obvious.

BORON

Between 1939 and 1944, several attempts to induce a boron deficiency in rats were unsuccessful, although the diets used apparently contained only 155–163 ng boron/g (9–11). In 1945, there was a report (12) that supplemental dietary boron enhanced survival and maintenance of body fat and elevated liver glycogen in potassium-deficient rats. Those findings were not confirmed in a subsequent study (13) in which rats were fed a different diet with an unknown boron content and different levels of boron supplementation.

After those reports, boron was generally accepted as being essential for plants, but not for animals. In 1981–1983, however, evidence was reported that indicated boron might be an essential nutrient (14,15). The evidence included depressed growth and abnormal bone development (similar to rickets) in boron-deprived (<0.2 $\mu g/g$ diet) chicks. Those signs of deprivation were more marked in chicks fed a cholecalciferol-deficient diet than in chicks fed a cholecalciferol-luxuriant diet. The findings indicated that boron and cholecalciferol interacted, but factorially arranged experiments using variable levels (deficient to luxuriant) of these nutrients did not show a statistically significant interaction. Subsequent factorially arranged experiments, using variable levels (deficient to luxuriant) of boron and magnesium, showed a statistical interaction between those two nutrients instead of boron and cholecalciferol. Boron deprivation signs of depressed growth, rachitic-like long bone histology, and elevated levels of alkaline phosphatase activity, magnesium and calcium in plasma were more marked when dietary magnesium was marginal (C. D. Hunt and F. H. Nielsen, unpublished observations).

At present, the evidence for essentiality of boron has come from studies done only in one laboratory and with one animal species—the chick. Thus, the establishment of boron as essential still requires further study. Findings to date should be confirmed in another laboratory, or by using another animal species. Meanwhile, suggestion of a possible dietary boron requirement for humans would be inappropriate. Nevertheless tablets containing magnesium carbonate and sodium borate are touted as a remedy for arthritis (16).

BROMINE

Only weak evidence suggests that bromine is an essential nutrient for animals. This evidence includes: (1) Bromide can substitute for part of the chloride requirement of chicks (17). (2) Trace amounts of dietary bromide elicited a small, but significant growth response in chicks and mice with hyperthyroid-induced depressed growth as a result of being fed a semi-synthetic diet containing iodinated casein (18,19).

In 1981, it was reported (20) that unusually low bromide concentrations occur in serum and brain of patients subjected to chronic hemodialysis; apparently the artificial kidney removed bromine. The bromine deficit was correlated with the insomnia exhibited by many hemodialysis patients. Subsequently, a double-blind trial was done in which either bromide or chloride was added to the dialysate of four patients on maintenance hemodialysis. Quality of sleep improved markedly in the two patients who received bromide, but not in those who received chloride. These findings are not the first association between bromide and quality of sleep. Before barbiturates were used, doctors prescribed bromide for sleep.

The limited findings to date do not show bromide is specifically required to prevent a suboptimal function. In the studies with animals, bromide apparently just replaced chloride or iodide. In the quality-of-sleep studies, bromide might have been acting pharmacologically. Thus, bromine cannot be considered an essential nutrient. Nevertheless, the findings indicate that the possible essentiality of bromine should be studied further. Bromine, however, is ubiquitous in the biosphere, and signs of deprivation might be hard to induce in experimental animals.

CADMIUM

The evidence, from two laboratories, suggesting that cadmium is an essential nutrient does not fulfill the definition of essentiality. Anke et al. (21) found in one experiment that, after 100 days of dietary treatment, growth was slower in goats fed 20 ng cadmium/g diet than in goats fed 250 ng cadmium/g diet. They stated, however, that their findings were inconclusive because the experiment was not repeated and two of five cadmium-deprived goats died from unknown causes. Schwarz and Spallholz (22) found that a dietary supplement of cadmium slightly stimulated growth of suboptimally growing rats but did not result in optimal growth. Apparently, the suboptimal growth was mainly due to riboflavin deficiency (22,23). It is unknown whether a deficiency of cadmium depresses growth in rats that are not riboflavin deficient. Criticisms of the experiments of Schwarz and Spallholz (22) are also reported in the discussion of tin (see below). Because findings did not show that cadmium deficiency consistently impaired any function of animals, cadmium cannot be considered an essential nutrient at this time.

FLUORINE

The beneficial function of fluoride in preventing human dental caries was discovered in the late 1930s. Subsequently, epidemiologic findings suggested that fluoride is beneficial for the maintenance of a normal skeleton in adults. A recent review (24) summarized those findings and a number of reports that described the treatment response of patients, suffering from osteoporosis and other demineralizing diseases, who were given substantial amounts of sodium fluoride. In some patients, back pain, bone density, and calcium balance were improved.

In the early 1970s, scientists suggested that fluoride is necessary for hematopoiesis, fertility, and growth in mice and rats. The suggestion, however, was based on experiments in which animals were not fed optimal diets. Schwarz and Milne (25) reported that a dietary supplement of fluoride slightly improved the growth of suboptimally growing rats but did not result in optimal growth. The shortcomings of that study were the same as those described for cadmium (see above) and tin (see below). Messer et al. (26) fed a marginally iron-deficient diet when they showed that high dietary fluoride (50 mg/liter of drinking water) improved hematopoiesis and fertility in mice. Subsequent studies showed that very high levels of dietary fluoride can improve iron absorption or utilization from a diet that is marginally sufficient in iron (27,28). To date, most of the findings that often are accepted as evidence for fluoride essentiality reflect a pharmacologic, not physiologic, action of fluoride. That is, high levels of orally administered fluoride alleviated a disorder caused by something other than fluoride deficiency. If tooth mottling is evidence of toxicity, near toxic amounts of fluoride prevent tooth decay caused by bacterial plaque. Also, near toxic levels of fluoride are needed for preventive or therapeutic action against osteoporosis, which is believed by some authorities to be a disorder of calcium-phosphorus metabolism. Extremely high levels of fluoride, that is, 50 $\mu g/ml$ of drinking water, probably acted through a pharmacologic mechanism to overcome depressed hematopoiesis and impaired reproduction caused by a marginal iron status in mice.

Therefore, signs of fluoride deficiency have not been described for any animal, and there is no conclusive evidence that fluoride is an essential nutrient for animals or humans. Lack of evidence, however, does not mean an essential function will not be found in the future.

Because it is not known to be essential, there is no dietary requirement for fluoride. Still, fluoride must be recognized as a trace element with beneficial properties. Therefore, the Food and Nutrition Board of the National Research Council estimated adequate and safe daily intakes of 0.1 to 0.5 mg fluoride for infants less than 6 months of age, 0.2 to 1.0 mg for infants between 6 and 12 months, 0.5 to 1.0 mg for children between the ages of 1 and 3 years, 1.0 and 2.5 mg for children between the ages of 4 and 6 years, 1.5 to 2.5 mg for children from 7 years to adulthood, and 1.5 to 4.0 mg for adults (29). These levels were considered to be protective against dental caries and perhaps against osteoporosis. Tabulations of average fluoride intake show large variation—0.78 to 3.44 mg daily (30). The variation apparently is caused by differences in the consumption of fluoridated water and high-fluoride foods, such as seafoods (5 to 10 $\mu g/g$), tea (100 $\mu g/g$), and cereal grains (1 to 3 $\mu g/g$).

LEAD

Findings suggesting that lead is an essential nutrient have come from two laboratories. Schwarz (31) found that lead slightly improved the growth of suboptimally growing rats but did not result in optimal growth. In a series of reports summarized recently (32) Kirchgessner and Reichlmayr-Lais reported that lead deprivation resulted in depressed growth and hypochromic microcytic anemia in rats. Also, lead deprivation apparently disturbed iron metabolism, and altered the activities of several enzymes (e.g., catalase) and the levels of several metabolites in serum and liver (e.g., cholesterol).

Both studies on lead essentiality have shortcomings. The study of Schwarz (31) has the same faults as the studies on the essentiality of cadmium (see above) or tin (see below). In the study of Kirchgessner and Reichlmayr-Lais (32), the most convincing evidence came from only a small number of very young rats in one of three experiments. In the first experiment, weanling rats were fed diets containing either 45 ng or 1 μg lead/g. After 30 days, dietary lead had no effect on the growing rats (33). In the second experiment, the experimental diets were fed to weanling female rats that were allowed to reproduce. The only positive finding in this experiment was that hematopoiesis was slightly depressed in 21-day-old lead-deprived pups. However, neither the dams, nor the remainder of the pups killed at age 48 days, were affected by lead deprivation. In the third experiment, lead-deprived and supplemented rats were allowed to reproduce through two generations (32,34). The lead-deprived rats were fed either 18 ng (F_1 generation) or 30 ng (F_2 generation) of lead/g of diet. The primary evidence of lead essentiality was from eight lead-deprived and ten lead-supplemented F_1 female rats examined 17 days after weaning (age 38 days). Lead deprivation markedly depressed growth and disturbed iron metabolism in this selected group of rats. In the other F_1 pups examined at older ages, however, the apparent effects of lead deprivation on growth, hematopoiesis, and iron disappeared. In the F_2 generation, no pups, at any age, exhibited signs of lead deprivation as marked as those exhibited by the eight female F_1 pups. Upon reviewing the data, the following questions seem appropriate: (1) Why did lead deprivation, contrary to the expected trend, affect F_2 pups less severely than F_1 pups? (2) Why did lead deprivation have only a transitory effect on rats? Organisms generally require essential nutrients throughout their lifetimes. Possible answers suggested by Reichlmayr-Lais and Kirchgessner (34) to those questions were: (1) The lead-deficient diet fed to older and F_2 rats contained more lead than the lead-deficient diet fed to F_1 rats. (2) Older rats homeostatically adapted to low dietary lead. On the other hand, perhaps lead had a pharmacologic effect, like that described for fluoride (see above), on iron metabolism in young rats. The lack of sufficient data to conclusively answer the questions indicates that the role of lead in nutrition and health should be clarified in additional studies. Furthermore, until such studies are done, lead probably should not be considered essential.

LITHIUM

Findings suggesting lithium is an essential nutrient have come from two laboratories. Anke et al. (35) found that lithium deprivation (2–3 μg lithium/g diet) depressed growth, fertility, and longevity of goats. In O'Dell's laboratory (36,37), rats fed a low-lithium diet (5–15 ng/g) grew adequately, but fertility was depressed in F_2 and F_3 dams. In addition, the lithium content was depressed in testes, seminal vesicles, and epididymis. Lithium concentrations were relatively high in the pituitary and adrenal glands and remained constant through two generations regardless of dietary lithium. Thus, two independent studies, in which the same sign of lithium deprivation—depressed fertility—was induced in two animal species, indicate that lithium is an essential nutrient. Furthermore, analyses of tissues suggested that lithium might have a role in endocrine function. Interpretation of the findings, however, is confounded by the wide difference between the two studies in the lithium content of the deficient diets (2–3 μg/g versus 5–15 ng/g). Possibly, the difference could be explained either by species differences in lithium requirement, or by an error in lithium analyses. Although emerging evidence strongly suggests that lithium is essential, concerns about the lack of marked deprivation signs and the uncertainty of what constitutes a deficient diet preclude stating conclusively that lithium is an essential nutrient. Those concerns also prevent any discussion of possible human requirements.

NICKEL

Nickel deprivation in animals was first described in 1970. The early studies, however, were conducted under conditions that produced suboptimal growth in the experimental animals (1). Also, some of the reported signs of nickel deprivation were shown inconsistently. Retrospective review of the methodology used in those studies indicated that much of the inconsistency was probably related to variation in the iron status of, and environmental conditions for, the experimental animals. Thus, most of the early findings apparently represented nickel deficiency modified by dietary and environmental conditions.

Since 1975, diets and environments that allow optimal growth and survival of experimental animals have been used in studies of nickel nutrition and metabolism. Signs of nickel deprivation have been described for six species—chick, cow, goat, minipig, rat, and sheep. The signs of nickel deprivation for each of the six species have been listed in reviews (1,38,39). The most prominent and consistent signs are depressed growth and hematopoiesis, and changes in the levels of iron, copper, and zinc in liver.

Recently, research on nickel has attempted to identify the biological function of nickel. Recent findings indicate that nickel functions either as a cofactor or structural component in specific metalloenzymes, or as a bioligand cofactor facilitating the intestinal absorption of the ferric ion.

Development of the hypothesis that nickel functions as an enzyme cofactor or structural component has been stimulated by the discovery of several nickel-containing enzymes in plants and microorganisms. Urease from jack bean (*Canavalia ensiformis*) was the first natural nickel metalloenzyme discovered (40,41). Subsequently, ureases from several other plants and microorganisms were identified as nickel metalloenzymes (42).

In bacteria that derive energy from the conversion of H_2 to CH_4 (methanogenic bacteria) or H_2O (Knallgas bacteria), the hydrogenase involved contains nickel, or requires nickel for its synthesis (43–45). In the hydrogenases of *Methanobacterium bryantii* and the sulfate-reducing bacterium, *Desulfovibrio gigas*, a substantial amount of the nickel is in the Ni^{3+} state (44,46). LeGall et al. (46) suggested that redox-sensitive nickel is an important catalytic component of the *D. gigas* hydrogenase, and may represent the binding site for the substrate H_2.

Other recently discovered nickel metalloenzymes include: (1) component C of methyl coenzyme M methylreductase, which reduces CH_3-S-CoM to methane and HS-CoM in methanogenic bacteria (43,47); (2) a moiety with carbon monoxide dehydrogenase activity which is part of a multi-enzyme complex that catalyzes the reductive carboxylation of methyltetrahydrofolate to acetate in acetogenic bacteria (43).

The finding of nickel metalloenzymes in plants and microorganisms suggests that nickel may have a similar function in animals. Nickel can activate many enzymes in vitro, but a role as a specific cofactor for any animal enzyme has not been shown (42).

The hypothesis that nickel might function as a bioligand cofactor facilitating the intestinal absorption of Fe^{3+} has been supported by findings in rats that show interactions between nickel and iron depend upon the form of dietary iron. Nickel synergistically interacted with iron to affect hematopoiesis in rats fed dietary iron as ferric sulfate only, but not as a mixture of ferric and ferrous sulfates (42). Furthermore, when low levels of ferric sulfate only were fed, whole body retention of $^{59}Fe^{3+}$ was less in nickel-deprived, even though they were more anemic, than in nickel-supplemented rats, whereas $^{59}Fe^{2+}$ retention was not affected by dietary nickel (1,48).

The mechanism through which nickel enhances Fe^{3+} absorption is unclear. For absorption by the duodenum, Fe^{3+} must be complexed, or converted to the more soluble Fe^{2+} form. The idea that nickel might act in an enzyme mechanism that converts Fe^{3+} to Fe^{2+} for absorption is attractive because of the recent finding of redox-sensitive nickel in enzymes of microorganisms (see above). However, the possibility that nickel promotes the absorption of Fe^{3+} per se by enhancing its complexation to a molecule that can be absorbed cannot be overlooked.

Nickel is an essential nutrient. By extrapolation from animal data, it is reasonable to postulate that nickel is required by humans. Moreover, the nickel requirement of animals may give a general idea of the possible amount of nickel required by humans. For rats and chicks, the nickel requirement apparently is about 50 μg/kg of diet, or slightly less (1). Calculated from data for monogastric animals, a suggested dietary nickel requirement of humans would be near 50 μg/kg of diet or 16 μg/1000 kcal (1).

Limited studies indicate that the oral intake of nickel by humans ranges between 170 and 700 μg/day, which would be ample to meet the hypothetical nickel requirement (49,50). Diets based on foods of animal origin and fats may be low in nickel (51). Rich sources of nickel include chocolate, nuts, dried beans and peas, and grains (52–54).

Imaginative research is needed on the role of nickel in human nutrition, health, and disease. The findings that nickel affects the absorption and metabolism of iron, and that iron status affects nickel metabolism, should be especially helpful in defining situations in which nickel would have nutritional significance.

SILICON

Early studies describing signs of silicon deprivation in chicks and rats have been summarized (55). Most of the signs indicated aberrant metabolism of connective tissue and bone. Animals in early studies were fed crystalline amino acid diets that did not give optimal growth in controls. Carlisle (56,57) recently developed a semisynthetic, silicon-deficient diet that produces near optimal growth in chicks. With this diet, in contrast to amino acid diets, silicon deprivation did not affect chick growth or outward appearance but did affect connective tissue and bone. Abnormalities included skull structural abnormalities, associated with depressed collagen content in bone, and long bone abnormalities, characterized by small, poorly formed joints and defective endochondrial bone growth. Silicon-deficient chick tibiae exhibited depressed contents of articular cartilage, water, hexosamine, and collagen. Thus, although some of the early evidence for the essentiality of silicon may have been disputable because of the poor growth of the control animals, Carlisle's more recent findings clarify the issue.

Both the distribution of silicon in the organism and the effect of silicon deficiency on connective tissue form and composition support the view that silicon functions as a biological cross-linking agent and contributes to the architecture and resilience of connective tissue. The connective tissue components in which silicon apparently plays a fundamental role in the cross-linking mechanism are collagen (55–57), elastin (58), and mucopolysaccharide (59). Unfortunately, the actual role has not been identified yet.

Silicon is apparently involved in bone calcification (55); however, the exact mechanism remains unclear. Some findings suggest a catalytic function for silicon. On the other hand, the marked influence of silicon on collagen and mucopolysaccharide formation and structure suggests that the influence of silicon on bone calcification is an indirect consequence of changes in these bone matrix components. Support for the latter view is that, in silicon-deficient animals, the formation of organic matrix, whether cartilage or bone, is apparently affected more severely than the mineralization process (57).

Ample evidence indicates that silicon can be accepted as an essential nutrient. Though the essentiality of silicon was suggested more than 10 years ago, little is known about its nutritional requirements. The form needed and minimum requirement have not been ascertained for any animal, so nothing can be said about possible human requirements. To prevent deficiency signs, chicks were fed 100–200 μg silicon, as sodium silicate, per g of diet. This probably should not be accepted as a requirement level because Schwarz (58) reported that other silicon compounds were 5–10 times as effective, per atom of silicon, as the silicate in preventing nutritional deficiency.

Silicon is an ubiquitous element and is supplied by many foods, especially unrefined grains such as unpolished rice (60). Foods of animal origin, except skin (e.g., chicken), are relatively low in silicon (55). A human balance study indicated that the oral intake of silicon by humans could be about 21–46 mg/day (61).

More work is needed to clarify the consequences of silicon deficiency in animals and humans. This has not prevented speculation, reviewed by Carlisle (55), that silicon might be involved in several human disorders including atherosclerosis, osteoarthritis, hypertension, and the process of aging. Those speculations demonstrate the critical need for study of silicon nutrition, especially its role in the process of aging.

TIN

The only evidence in favor of tin essentiality is the report that tin added to an experimental diet slightly improved the growth of suboptimally growing, apparently riboflavin-deficient rats (23) but did not result in optimal growth (62). The use of riboflavin-deficient rats in tin essentiality studies is of particular concern because the oxidation-reduction potential of $Sn^{2+} \rightleftarrows Sn^{4+}$ is 0.13 v, which is near the oxidation-reduction potential of flavine enzymes. Attempts to show that tin deprivation depressed growth in riboflavin-adequate rats were unsuccessful, even though animals and dietary materials used were from the same sources as those used in the study with riboflavin-deficient rats (F. H. Nielsen, unpublished observations). Thus, it cannot be stated unequivocally that tin deprivation reproducibly impairs a function from optimal to suboptimal.

The study (62) that suggested the nutritional essentiality of tin can also be criticized as follows: (1) The growth difference between "deficient controls" and tin-supplemented rats (about 5—7 g after 25 to 30 days on experiment) may be of questionable physiologic meaning. Because it was so small, the response may have been an indication that tin prevented the breakdown of some essential nutrient (e.g., riboflavin), substituted for some trace element lacking in the diet, or acted as an antibiotic. Those possibilities suggest that the action of tin was pharmacologic, rather than physiologic. (2) The addition of tin to the diet was of no apparent benefit to deficient-control animals in subsequent studies. For example, the deficient-control gained about 1.3—1.9 g/day; tin supplemented rats, 1.7—2.2 g/day. However, even with the addition of tin, and some other possibly essential elements such as fluorine, to the same diet (25), the deficient-controls in a lead essentiality study (31) still gained only 1.5—2.1 g/day, and lead-supplemented rats, 1.6—2.2 g/day. Subsequent to the lead study, deficient-controls and cadmium-supplemented rats exhibited similar daily weight gains (22). The finding that deficient-controls gained at the same rate in each study (tin, fluorine, lead, and cadmium) was unexplained, even though the deficient-controls would be expected to grow better in the latter studies because their diets contained additional "essential" elements.

Without more conclusive evidence, tin should not be considered an essential trace element. Moreover, the description of a hypothetical biological function or nutritional requirement would be inappropriate.

VANADIUM

The essentiality of vanadium is difficult to categorize because reported evidence, reviewed recently (42), is inconsistent. Basically, several groups found in many experiments that vanadium deprivation adversely affected growth, feathering, hematocrits, plasma cholesterol, bone development, and liver lipid, phospholipid, and cholesterol content in chicks, as well as perinatal survival, growth, physical appearance, hematocrits, plasma cholesterol, and liver lipid and phospholipid content in rats. Unfortunately, no sign of vanadium deprivation in either chicks or rats was found consistently throughout all experiments.

Apparently, the inconsistency of vanadium deprivation signs was related to the fact that vanadium metabolism is sensitive to changes in the composition of the diet (38). Shuler and Nielsen (63) suggested that the iron and cystine status of experimental animals must be controlled if findings from different studies of vanadium nutrition are to be compared. In moderately iron-deficient rats, for example, vanadium deprivation depressed hematocrit when dietary cystine was 4.65 mg/g, and elevated hematocrit when dietary cystine was 10.15 mg/g. Vanadium deprivation did not affect hematocrit in rats fed adequate iron.

Differences in levels of dietary cystine (perhaps amino acid composition in general) and iron may explain some of the inconsistencies in vanadium deprivation signs found in earlier studies. Strasia (64) found that vanadium deprivation depressed growth and elevated hematocrits in rats when he fed a diet that contained 20 μg iron/g and 269 g vitamin-free casein/kg. On the other hand, Williams (65) found that vanadium deprivation did not affect growth and hematocrits when a diet containing 35 μg iron/g and 175 g vitamin-free casein/kg was fed. Possibly those differences in iron and protein levels were large enough to account for the differences between these two studies. Similar comparisons could be made for the studies of Hopkins and Mohr (66,67), Schwarz and Milne (68), and Nielsen et al. (69).

Recently, interest in vanadium has been aroused by the finding in vitro that vanadate (vanadium in the 5+ state) is a potent inhibitor of (Na,K)-ATPase and other phosophoryl-transfer enzymes. Vanadium is present in tissues at concentrations that might inhibit phosphoryl-transfer enzymes in vivo. Therefore, Macara (70) hypothesized that vanadium functions in vivo as a regulator of (Na,K)-ATPase, and thus the sodium pump. The proposal of a regulatory function for vanadium would be strengthened by evidence of an in vivo mechanism whereby vanadium, which apparently exists in tissue as the relatively inactive 4+ oxidation state complexed to protein or small molecules, would be converted to vanadium in the 5+ state. The studies suggesting a regulatory function for vanadium are more completely summarized elsewhere (1,42).

Failure to define the conditions that induce reproducible deficiency in animals has prevented the establishment of vanadium essentiality, but emerging evidence suggests that vanadium will be found essential for animals and humans. Findings to date can only allude to a possible vanadium requirement. Diets containing 4–25 ng vanadium/g adversely affect rats and chicks under certain conditions (38). Apparently any human requirement for vanadium would be very small.

The vanadium content of most foods is low (49,71,72), generally not more than a few ng/g. Myron et al. (49) found that nine institutional diets supplied 12.4–30.1 μg of vanadium daily, and intake averaged 20 μg. Byrne and Kosta (72) stated that the daily dietary intake of vanadium is on the order of a few tens of μg and may vary widely. Since food contains very little vanadium, and vanadium metabolism apparently is profoundly affected by other dietary components, there is a possibility that vanadium intake is not always optimal. That possibility demonstrates the need to clarify the biological function of vanadium, the conditions that produce vanadium deficiency, and the dietary components and their mechanisms that affect vanadium metabolism.

CONCLUDING REMARKS

Knowledge about the physiologic functions and optimum intakes of the ultratrace elements that have been identified as essential (arsenic, nickel, and silicon) should be extended and refined. Further research might establish essentiality for some or all of the other eight proposed ultratrace elements and might even identify new candidates. The research might also reveal that some ultratrace elements are more important in human health than is now generally acknowledged. Those who are concerned with human nutrition should be cognizant of this possibility, and therefore should not consider the ultratrace elements as esoteric when considering the adequacy of diets. However, the consumption of a varied diet composed of many different foods increases the probability of an adequate supply of all essential micronutrients, including the ultratrace elements.

REFERENCES

1. F.H. Nielsen, Possible future implications of nickel, arsenic, silicon, vanadium, and other ultratrace elements in human nutrition. In A.S. Prasad, ed., *Clinical, Biochemical, and Nutritional Aspects of Trace Elements, Current Topics in Nutrition and Disease,* Vol. 6, Alan R. Liss, New York, 1982, p. 379.

2. F.H Nielsen and E.O. Uthus, Arsenic. In E. Frieden, ed., *Biochemistry of the Essential Ultra-Trace Elements,* Plenum, New York, in press.

3. E.O. Uthus, W.E. Cornatzer, and F.H. Nielsen, Consequences of arsenic deprivation in laboratory animals. In W.H. Lederer and R.J. Fensterheim, eds., *Arsenic: Industrial, Biomedical, Environmental Perspectives,* Van Nostrand Reinhold, New York, 1983, p. 173.

4. W.E. Cornatzer, E.O. Uthus, J.A. Haning, and F.H. Nielsen, Effect of arsenic deprivation on phosphatidylcholine biosynthesis in liver microsomes on the rat. *Nutr. Reports Int.* **27,** 821 (1983).

5. M. Anke, M. Grün, M. Partschefeld, B. Groppel, and A. Hennig, Essentiality and function of arsenic. In M. Kirchgessner, ed., *Trace Element Metabolism in Man and Animals-3,* Tech. Univ. München, Freising-Weihenstephan, 1978, p. 248.

6. H.A. Schroeder and J.J. Balassa, Abnormal trace metals in man: Arsenic. *J. Chronic Dis.* **19,** 85 (1966).

7. C.F. Jelinek and P.E. Corneliussen, Levels of arsenic in the United States food supply. *Environ. Health Perspect.* **19,** 83 (1977).

8. S. Horiguchi, K. Teramoto, T. Kurono, and K. Ninomiya, The arsenic, copper, lead, manganese and zinc contents of daily foods and beverages in Japan and the estimate of their daily intake. *Osaka City Med. J.* **24,** 131 (1978).

9. E. Hove, C.A. Elvehjem, and E.B. Hart, Boron in animal nutrition. *Am. J. Physiol.* **127,** 689 (1939).

10. E. Orent-Keiles, The role of boron in the diet of the rat. *Proc. Soc. Exp. Biol. Med.* **44,** 199 (1941).

11. J.D. Teresi, E. Hove, C.A. Elvehjem, and E.B. Hart, Further study of boron in the nutrition of rat. *Am. J. Physiol.* **140,** 513 (1944).

12. J.T. Skinner and J.S. McHargue, Response of rats to boron supplements when fed rations low in potassium. *Am. J. Physiol.* **143,** 385 (1945).

13. R.H. Follis, Jr., The effect of adding boron to a potassium-deficient diet in the rat. *Am. J. Physiol.* **150,** 520 (1947).

14. C.D. Hunt and F.H. Nielsen, Interaction between boron and cholecalciferol in the chick. In J.McC. Howell, J.M. Gawthorne, and C.L. White, eds., *Trace Element Metabolism in Man and Animals,* Vol. 4, Australian Academy of Science, Canberra, 1981, p. 597.

15. C.D. Hunt and F.H. Nielsen, Dietary boron affects calcium metabolism. *Fed. Proc.* **42,** 398 (1983).

16. R.E. Newnham, Mineral imbalance and boron deficiency. In J.McC. Howell, J.M. Gawthorne, and C.L. White, eds., *Trace Element*

Metabolism in Man and Animals, Vol. 4, Australian Academy of Science, Canberra, 1981, p. 400.

17. R. M. Leach, Jr. and M. C. Nesheim, Studies on chloride deficiency in chicks. *J. Nutr.* **81**, 193 (1963).

18. J. W. Huff, D. K. Bosshardt, O. P. Miller, and R. H. Barnes, A nutritional requirement for bromine. *Proc. Soc. Exp. Biol. Med.* **92**, 216 (1956).

19. D. K. Bosshardt, J. W. Huff, and R. H. Barnes, Effect of bromine on chick growth. *Proc. Soc. Exp. Biol. Med.* **92**, 219 (1956).

20. P. L. Oe, R. D. Vis, J. H. Meijer, F. van Langevelde, W. Allon, C. v. d. Meer, and H. Verheul, Bromine deficiency and insomnia in patients on dialysis. In J. McC. Howell, J. M. Gawthorne, and C. L. White, eds., *Trace Element Metabolism in Man and Animals*, Vol. 4, Australian Academy of Science, Canberra, 1981, p. 526.

21. M. Anke, A. Hennig, B. Groppel, M. Partschefeld, and M. Grün, The biochemical role of cadmium. In M. Kirchgessner, ed., *Trace Element Metabolism in Man and Animals-3*, Tech. Univ. München, Freising-Weihenstephan, 1978, p. 540.

22. K. Schwarz and J. E. Spallholz, The potential essentiality of cadmium. In F. Bolck, M. Anke, and H.-J. Schneider, eds., *Kadmium-Symposium*, Friedrich-Schiller-Universität, Jena, 1979, p. 188.

23. J. K. Moran and K. Schwarz, Light sensitivity of riboflavin in amino acid diets. *Fed. Proc.* **37**, 671 (1978).

24. S. A. Anderson, *Effects of Certain Vitamins and Minerals on Calcium and Phosphorus Homeostasis*, LSRO, Fed. Amer. Soc. Exp. Biol., Bethesda, 1982, 93 pp.

25. K. Schwarz and D. B. Milne, Fluorine requirement for growth in rats. *Bioinorg. Chem.* **1**, 331 (1972).

26. H. H. Messer, W. D. Armstrong, and L. Singer, Essentiality and function of fluoride. In W. G. Hoekstra, J. W. Suttie, H. E. Ganther, and W. Mertz, eds., *Trace Element Metabolism in Animals-2*, University Park, Baltimore, 1974, p. 425.

27. S. Tao and J. W. Suttie, Evidence for a lack of an effect of dietary fluoride level on reproduction in mice. *J. Nutr.* **106**, 1115 (1976).

28. M. E. Wegner, L. Singer, R. H. Ophaug, and S. G. Magil, The interrelation of fluoride and iron in anemia. *Proc. Soc. Exp. Biol. Med.* **153**, 414 (1976).

29. Committee on Dietary Allowances, Food and Nutrition Board, National Research Council. *Recommended Dietary Allowances*, 9th ed., National Academy of Sciences, Washington, D.C., 1980.

30. L. Kramer, D. Osis, E. Wiatrowski, and H. Spencer, Dietary fluoride in different areas in the United States. *Am. J. Clin. Nutr.* **27**, 590 (1974).

31. K. Schwarz, Potential essentiality of lead. *Arh. Hig. Rada Toksikol.* (*Suppl. — Internat. Symp. Environ. Lead Res.*) **26**, 13 (1975).

32. M. Kirchgessner and A. M. Reichlmayr-Lais, Lead deficiency and its effects on growth and metabolism. In J. McC. Howell, J. M. Gawthorne, and C. L. White, eds., *Trace Element Metabolism in Man and Animals*, Vol.

4, Australian Academy of Science, Canberra, 1981, p. 390.

33. A. M. Reichlmayr-Lais and M. Kirchgessner, Depletionsstudien zur Essentialität von Blei an wachsenden Ratten. *Arch. Tierernaehr.* **31**, 731 (1981).

34. A. M. Reichlmayr-Lais and M. Kirchgessner, Hämatologische Veränderungen im alimentären Blei-Mangel. *Ann. Nutr. Metab.* **25**, 281 (1981).

35. M. Anke, M. Grün, B. Groppel, and H. Kronemann, The biological importance of lithium. In M. Anke and H.-J. Schneider, eds., *Mengen- und Spuren-elemente*, Karl-Marx Universität, Leipzig, 1981, p. 217.

36. J. Burt, R. P. Dowdy, E. E. Pickett, and B. L. O'Dell, Effect of low dietary lithium on tissue lithium content in rats. *Fed. Proc.*, **41**, 460 (1982).

37. E. L. Patt, E. E. Pickett, and B. L. O'Dell, Effect of dietary lithium levels on tissue lithium concentrations, growth rate, and reproduction in the rat. *Bioinorg. Chem.* **9**, 299 (1978).

38. F. H. Nielsen, Evidence of the essentiality of arsenic, nickel and vanadium and their possible nutritional significance. In H. H. Draper, ed., *Advances in Nutritional Research*, Vol. 3, Plenum, New York, 1980, p. 157.

39. F. H. Nielsen, Nickel. In E. Frieden, ed., *Biochemistry of the Essential Ultra-Trace Elements*, Plenum, New York, in press.

40. N. E. Dixon, R. L. Blakeley, and B. Zerner, Jack bean urease (EC 3.5.1.5). III. The involvement of active-site nickel ion in inhibition by β-mercaptoethanol, phosphoramidate, and fluoride. *Can. J. Biochem.* **58**, 481 (1980).

41. N. E. Dixon, C. Gazzola, C. J. Asher, D. S. W. Lee, R. L. Blakeley, and B. Zerner, Jack bean urease (EC 3.5.1.5). II. The relationship between nickel, enzymatic activity, and the "abnormal" ultraviolet spectrum. The nickel content of jack beans. *Can. J. Biochem.* **58**, 474 (1980).

42. F. H. Nielsen, Possible functions and medical significance of the abstruse trace elements. In A. E. Martell, ed., *Inorganic Chemistry in Biology and Medicine*, ACS Symposium Series 140, American Chemical Society, Washington, D.C., 1980, p. 23.

43. R. K. Thauer, G. Diekert, and P. Schönheit, Biological role of nickel. *Trends Biochem. Sci. (Pers. Ed.)* **5**, 304 (1980).

44. J. R. Lancaster, Jr., New biological paramagnetic center: Octahedrally coordinated nickel(III) in the methanogenic bacteria. *Science* **216**, 1324 (1982).

45. C. D. P. Partridge and M. G. Yates, Effect of chelating agents on hydrogenase in *Azotobacter chroococcum.* Evidence that nickel is required for hydrogenase synthesis. *Biochem. J.* **204**, 339 (1982).

46. J. LeGall, P. O. Ljungdahl, I. Moura, H. D. Peck, Jr., A. V. Xavier, J. J. G. Moura, M. Teixera, B. H. Huynh, and D. V. Der Vartanian, The presence of redox-sensitive nickel in the periplasmic hydrogenase from *Desulfovibrio gigas. Biochem. Biophys. Res. Commun.* **106**, 610 (1982).

47. W. L. Ellefson, W. B. Whitman, and R. S. Wolfe, Nickel-containing factor F_{430}: Chromophore of the methylreductase of methanobacterium. *Biochemistry* **79**, 3707 (1982).
48. F. H. Nielsen, Nickel deprivation in the rat: Effect on the absorption of ferric ions. In M. Anke, H.-J. Schneider, and C. Brückner, eds., *3. Spurenelement - Symposium Nickel*, Friedrich-Schiller-Universität, Jena, 1980, p. 33.
49. D. R. Myron, T. J. Zimmerman, T. R. Shuler, L. M. Klevay, D. E. Lee, and F. H. Nielsen, Intake of nickel and vanadium by humans. A survey of selected diets. *Am. J. Clin. Nutr.* **31**, 527 (1978).
50. G. K. Murthy, U. S. Rhea, and J. T. Peeler, Levels of copper, nickel, vanadium, and strontium in institutional total diets. *Environ. Sci. Tech.* **7**, 1042 (1973).
51. H. A. Schroeder, J. J. Balassa, and I. H. Tipton, Abnormal trace metals in man—nickel. *J. Chron. Dis.* **15**, 51 (1962).
52. G. Ellen, G. van den Bosch-Tibbesma, and F. F. Douma, Nickel content of various Dutch foodstuffs. *Z. Lebensm. Unters.-Forsch.* **166**, 145 (1978).
53. A. K. Furr, L. H. MacDaniels, L. E. St. John, Jr., W. H. Gutenman, I. S. Pakkola, and D. J. Lisk, Elemental composition of tree nuts. *Bull. Environ. Contam. Toxicol.* **21**, 392 (1979).
54. H. Kronemann, M. Anke, S. Thomas, and E. Redel, The nickel concentration of different food- and feed-stuffs—from areas with and without nickel exposure. In M. Anke, H.-J. Schneider, and C. Brückner, eds., *3. Spurenelement—Symposium Nickel*, Friedrich-Schiller-Universität, Jena, GDR, 1980, p. 221.
55. E. M. Carlisle, Silicon. *Nutr. Rev.* **33**, 257 (1975).
56. E. M. Carlisle, A silicon requirement for normal skull formation in chicks. *J. Nutr.* **110**, 352 (1980).
57. E. M. Carlisle, Biochemical and morphological changes associated with long bone abnormalities in silicon deficiency. *J. Nutr.* **110**, 1046 (1980).
58. K. Schwarz, Recent dietary trace element research, exemplified by tin, fluorine, and silicon. *Fed. Proc.*, **33**, 1748 (1974).
59. J. Loeper, J. Loeper, and M. Fragny, The physiological role of the silicon and its antiatheromatous action. *Nobel Symp. 1977* **40**, 281 (1978).
60. B. M. Kennedy and M. Schelstraete, A note on silicon in rice endosperm. *Cereal Chem.* **52**, 854 (1975).
61. J. L. Kelsay, K. M. Behall, and E. S. Prather, Effect of fiber from fruits and vegetables on metabolic responses of human subjects. II. Calcium, magnesium, iron and silicon balances. *Am. J. Clin. Nutr.* **32**, 1876 (1979).
62. K. Schwarz, D. B. Milne, and E. Vinyard, Growth effects of tin compounds in rats maintained in a trace element-controlled environment. *Biochem. Biophys. Res. Commun.* **40**, 22 (1970).
63. T. R. Shuler and F. H. Nielsen, Interactions among vanadium, iron, and cystine in rats: Liver content of selected trace elements. *Proc. N.D. Acad. Sci.* **37**, 88 (1983).

64. C. A. Strasia, *Vanadium: Essentiality and Toxicity in the Laboratory Rat.* Ph.D. thesis, Purdue University, 1971, 49 pp.

65. D. L. Williams, *Biological Value of Vanadium for Rats, Chickens, and Sheep.* Ph.D. thesis, Purdue University, 1973, 98 pp.

66. L. L. Hopkins, Jr. and H. E. Mohr, The biological essentiality of vanadium. In W. Mertz and W. E. Cornatzer, eds., *Newer Trace Elements in Nutrition,* Dekker, New York, 1971, p. 195.

67. L. L. Hopkins, Jr. and H. E. Mohr, Vanadium as an essential nutrient. *Fed. Proc.,* **33,** 1773 (1974).

68. K. Schwarz and D. B. Milne, Growth effects of vanadium in the rat. *Science* **174,** 426 (1971).

69. F. H. Nielsen, D. R. Myron, and E. O. Uthus, Newer trace elements— vanadium (V) and arsenic (As) deficiency signs and possible metabolic roles. In M. Kirchgessner, ed., *Trace Element Metabolism in Man and Animals-3,* Tech. Univ. München, Freising-Weihenstephan, 1978, p. 244.

70. I. G. Macara, Vanadium—an element in search of a role. *Trends Biochem. Sci. (Pers. Ed.)* **5,** 92 (1980).

71. D. R. Myron, S. H. Givand, and F. H. Nielsen, Vanadium content of selected foods as determined by flameless atomic absorption spectroscopy. *Agric. Food Chem.* **25,** 297 (1977).

72. A. R. Byrne and L. Kosta, Vanadium in foods and in human body fluids and tissues. *Sci. Total Environ.* **10,** 17 (1978).

Special Foods and Diets

7

Vegetarianism and Health

TERRY D. SHULTZ, Ph.D.
Associate Professor of Nutrition
Department of Nutrition
School of Public Health
and
Assistant Professor of Biochemistry
Department of Biochemistry
School of Medicine

WINSTON J. CRAIG, Ph.D., R.D.
Associate Professor of Nutrition

PATRICIA K. JOHNSTON, M.S., M.P.H., R.D.
Assistant Professor of Nutrition

ALBERT SANCHEZ, Dr.P.H., R.D.
Professor of Nutrition

U.D. REGISTER, Ph.D., R.D.
Professor and Chairman of Nutrition
Department of Nutrition
School of Public Health
Loma Linda University
Loma Linda, California

Address correspondence to Terry D. Shultz, Ph.D., Associate Professor, Department of Nutrition, School of Public Health, Loma Linda University, Loma Linda, California 92350.

ABSTRACT

Vegetarianism has been practiced for centuries. Present-day vegetarians have chosen this dietary practice for a variety of reasons: philosophical orientation, spiritual outlook, health considerations, or ecological concerns. The "new" vegetarians are of special interest because their food habits differ from those of more traditional vegetarians, such as the Seventh-Day Adventists (SDAs). The most restrictive total vegetarian diets (e.g., Zen macrobiotic) may be hazardous to nutritional status and general health, particularly during pregnancy, lactation, and childhood. However, as the diet becomes less restrictive, the ability to meet nutritional requirements increases, and vegetarian diets, if carefully planned, are nutritionally adequate. A knowledge of food composition and basic nutrition principles underlies the achievement of optimal nutrient intake in this or any other diet. A well-balanced lacto- or lacto-ovo-vegetarian diet is recommended for those who wish to follow a vegetarian regimen. This is an appropriate intermediate step for those who want to adopt a total vegetarian diet. There is increasing evidence to suggest that the vegetarian diet may be the diet of choice for the prevention and treatment of various diseases. However, more research is needed to identify those elements in the vegetarian diet that may be associated with increased health benefits.

INTRODUCTION

According to the biblical record, mankind's first diet was of plant origin (Genesis 1:29 and 2:18). The history of the rise and wane of the vegetarian lifestyle was published by Hardinge and Crooks (1). During the last 20 years there has been a resurgence of interest in vegetarianism for a variety of reasons. Ecological, philosophical, and religious concerns motivated many persons. Perhaps the largest number have made the change from omnivorous to vegetarian diets for reasons of health. Wide publicity has been given to numerous epidemiological studies which show that a high intake of animal foods is associated with increased incidence of cardiovascular disease, cancer of the breast and colon, and other diseases. By contrast, a vegetarian diet (or an omnivorous diet of much-reduced animal content), is associated with lower risk of these diseases. The United States Dietary Goals and Dietary Guidelines encourage the use of more plant foods and fewer fatty animal foods as a means of improving the health of all Americans. Scientific evidence of the nutritional adequacy of a properly planned vegetarian diet has given further stimulus to the shift from an omnivorous to a vegetarian lifestyle. Poorly planned vegetarian diets, like inadequately formulated omnivorous diets, can lead to nutritional deficiencies. Sound nutritional principles are required in planning any diet. This report presents information regarding the vegetarian diet, its possible problems, its health implications, and guidelines regarding its use. Recent and related information on the subject has been published elsewhere (2–5).

Vegetarian Diets

The term "vegetarian" is often applied loosely to persons on a wide variety of diets and therefore needs further clarification. Total vegetarians (TVs) are persons who eat only plant foods. Their diets usually include vegetables, fruits, whole grain breads and cereals, peas, beans, other legumes, nuts, and seeds. Some use soy milk and meat analogs. They exclude all meat, poultry, fish, eggs, and dairy products. Some TVs, such as those known as vegans, may restrict their use of certain plant foods and avoid contact with any animal product, including leather, which requires the slaughter of animals.

Lacto-vegetarians (LVs) are persons who use milk and other dairy products in addition to plant foods. Lacto-ovo-vegetarians (LOVs) add eggs to their diets. Some individuals exclude meat but use fish (pescovegetarians) or poultry (pollovegetarians).

The "new" vegetarians are mostly young adults who emerged in the United States since 1960. They follow the diet and lifestyle of several philosophical or religious groups heavily influenced by Eastern thought. The "new" vegetarians are quite diverse: some use fish and poultry, others are LOVs, a good proportion are total vegetarians. Within the last group are some who abstain from one or more foods, including cereals, grains, legumes, fruits, processed or cooked foods, or foods not organically grown. Some of these individuals follow extreme and unsound nutritional principles (e.g., extremes in the Zen macrobiotic diet) and are at some risk of severe nutritional deficiencies. (References 2–5 provide a more complete discussion of types of vegetarians.)

NUTRITIONAL ADEQUACY

Adulthood

Vegetarianism has gained an unprecedented popularity in recent years; we feel that the shift from a typical Western diet to an LV or LOV diet does much to promote good health. Register and Sonnenberg (6) have concluded that adequate amounts of essential nutrients can be provided by vegetarian diets; the general nutritional adequacy of vegetarian diets has been documented by others (7–10). Restrictive or ill-planned vegetarian diets, however, may compromise nutritional adequacy.

The recommended daily protein intake is 56 g for men and 44 g for women at approximate calorie levels of 2700 and 2000, respectively. These recommendations represent diets that contain 8–9% of the calories as protein. Many plant and animal foods equal or exceed this protein-to-calorie concentration (e.g., potato, 8%; wheat, 13%; beans, 23%; broccoli, 35%; and milk, 23%). Hardinge and Stare (7) reported that self-selected diets of plant origin generally exceeded these recommendations. They found that omnivorous adult men and women had daily intakes of 125 and 94 g of protein, LOVs consumed 98 and 82 g, while TVs were ingesting 83 and 61 g of protein, respectively. Diets including only plant proteins contained 10% of the calories as protein. Thus, a vegetarian diet adequate in calories can easily exceed present-day protein recommendations, and the quantity of protein need not be of central concern.

Early studies reported that optimal protein utilization required all the essential amino acids to be present in the correct proportions. This finding was derived from studies where one or more amino acids were totally absent from the diet. However, it has been reported (11) that a meal low in (but not devoid of) an essential amino acid may be supplemented by adding the limiting amino acid at a subsequent meal, a principle known as delayed time supplementation. These studies have cast doubt on the necessity of simultaneous intake of complementary proteins *in vivo*. At one time, proteins were classified as complete or incomplete. This idea was based on studies of protein derived from single foods fed as sole protein sources. It is unrealistic to categorize single foods in this way, since protein quality depends on the total amino acid composition of a meal and not whether the diet contains individual foods that are incomplete or complete protein sources.

Some of us have studied the complementary value of vegetable and animal protein combinations in individual meals and weekly diets. Sanchez et al. (12,13) found that ideal combinations of protein quality were achieved when cereal-based diets were supplemented with ¼ to⅓of the protein from legumes. The protein quality of these combinations was equivalent to those of combinations of cereal diets with animal protein. The quality of vegetable proteins may thus be improved by combining with complementary proteins (animal or vegetable) in the same or subsequent meals. The result, either way, will provide essential amino acids in the amount and proportion needed to perform the essential functions of tissue building and maintenance. Hardinge et al. (14) have shown that vegetarian diets provide an adequate supply of the essential amino acids.

Individuals living in developed countries are unlikely to become deficient in any essential amino acid unless they adopt bizarre diets or severely restrict their dietary intake. It is of course good practice to include some protein at each meal. The American Dietetic Association states (3):

In order to achieve good protein nutrition, scientific studies and human experience tend to show that meticulous measuring and mixing is not crucial. Rather the emphasis is on choosing a wide assortment of as unrefined foods as practical and planning balanced meals for the day rather than juggling food items to effect precise balance for each meal.

The intake of certain nutrients may be marginal in some restricted vegetarian diets. This depends on the extent of the restrictions. Vegan diets may, in the absence of dairy foods, be low in calcium and riboflavin. Brown and Bergan (9) found the nutrient intakes of 50 well-educated young adult Zen macrobiotic followers to be insufficient in calories, calcium, and riboflavin, and in iron among women. Similarly, Shultz and Leklem (15) found lower dietary intake of energy, riboflavin, calcium, iron, and vitamin B-6 among groups of Seventh-Day Adventist (SDA) vegetarian and nonvegetarian women. The low iron and vitamin B-6 intakes are of concern to both vegetarian and nonvegetarian women. Vegetarian women could easily supplement their iron and vitamin B-6 intakes by increasing their consumption of cereals, legumes, nuts, and green leafy vegetables. Monsen et al. (16) have shown in human studies that ascorbic acid increases iron absorption; if foods high in ascorbic acid were consumed together with foods high in iron, iron reserves could be enhanced. The TV needs to give special attention to adequate intakes of calcium, riboflavin, and vitamin D, supplied in nonvegetarian diets largely by milk and milk products. Other calcium sources include dark green leafy vegetables, almonds, filberts, sesame seeds, legumes, fortified soy milk, and tofu. Good dietary sources of riboflavin are milk and milk products, dark green leafy vegetables, legumes, and whole grains. Inadequate dietary calcium may be compounded by insufficient intake of vitamin D, which is important for optimal calcium absorption. Vitamin D occurs naturally in only a few foods of animal origin, such as egg yolk, butter, liver, and fish. Some foods are fortified with vitamin D; the major dietary source for Americans is fortified milk. Wherever dietary sources of vitamin D are minimal and exposure to sunshine is limited, supplementation is appropriate. However, it should be emphasized that excessive amounts of vitamins A and D are potentially harmful; supplementation, if used, should be as suggested by the Recommended Dietary Allowances (RDA).

Total vegetarians eat no food of animal origin. They are of interest with respect to international issues regarding long-range food production. Additionally, their dietary habits may offer valuable clues as to whether a vegan diet can be nutritionally adequate for maintaining health. Several studies (17,18) have reported that the health status of vegans was not different from that of subjects consuming a nonvegetarian diet. Low serum vitamin B-12 levels have been reported in vegetarians (19,20), although clinical symptoms of deficiency are rare. Normal blood formation and mental functions can be maintained at low serum levels over an extended length of time; however, vitamin B-12 deficiencies may occur at wide-ranging levels. Because they are such good sources of vitamin B-12 and other nutrients, the consumption of milk and milk products is to be encouraged. For persons to whom dairy products are unacceptable, fortified soymilk or fortified vegetable protein analogs may well be suggested. It should be noted that some persons following the more restrictive diets are unaware of the importance of this vitamin; some of the same persons may be reluctant to seek medical care. When they do seek medical advice they should be approached with respect, sensitivity, and diplomacy in order to facilitate their compliance with suggestions for an improved nutritional status.

Pregnancy, Lactation, and Growth

Pregnancy, lactation, and periods of rapid growth are times of special concern for the adequacy of nutrient intake regardless of a person's dietary lifestyle. However, several nutrients may be of particular interest to the vegetarian, depending on which foods are excluded from the diet.

Vegetarians, especially those who follow the more restrictive patterns, have been found to weigh appreciably less than their nonvegetarian counterparts; such women may enter pregnancy at less than ideal body weight (7). Since pre-pregnancy weight and weight gain during pregnancy are both associated with pregnancy outcome, these factors are of particular importance to pregnant vegetarian women.

Few studies have looked at pregnancy outcomes among vegetarian women. Hardinge and Stare (7) found no difference in complications or the average weight gain between LOV and nonvegetarian women. The average birthweights and lengths of infants of the two groups did not differ statistically; however, the mean birthweight of infants born to nonvegetarian women tended to be slightly more than that of infants born to vegetarian women. A recent study of the health of vegans during pregnancy found no statistical difference in birthweights, live births, miscarriages, toxemia, or congenital malformations as compared to their nonvegetarian controls (21). Breast feeding was significantly more prevalent among the vegetarians (95% versus 31%) (21). A study reported by Shull et al. (22) found no difference in reported birthweights between macrobiotic and nonmacrobiotic vegetarian male infants; however, a greater proportion of female macrobiotic infants had birthweights less than one standard deviation below the mean. In the study, all infants with birthweights less than 2500 grams were macrobiotic. Similarly, Dwyer et al. (23) reported that macrobiotic girls weighed significantly less at birth than other vegetarians. These findings suggest a possible adverse effect on pregnancy outcome of a restrictive dietary intake.

Protein intake may be of particular concern because of possible low energy intake due to a low-caloric-density, high-fiber diet that may exclude animal products. It should be noted that whenever energy intake is limiting, protein will be used for energy instead of for tissue synthesis. Attention should be given to meeting both quantitative (an additional 30 g) and qualitative protein needs during pregnancy.

Vitamin and mineral needs are increased during pregnancy and are important in both vegetarian and nonvegetarian diets. Iron supplements are frequently prescribed during pregnancy; however, vegetarian women who do not seek medical advice should be cognizant of good dietary sources. Emphasis should also be placed on consumption at each meal of foods high in ascorbic acid, thus enhancing the availability of iron. Some concern has been expressed regarding the bioavailability of zinc in vegetarian diets, especially during pregnancy, since zinc deficiency has been associated with various congenital malformations.

Although studies comparing LOV and nonvegetarian pregnant women show no difference in their zinc status (24,25), care should be taken to assure an adequate intake.

There are no practical plant food sources for vitamin B-12, and deficiency during infancy can have serious and irreversible consequences. Such deficiencies have been reported in recent years with increasing frequency (26–28). The symptoms of fretfulness, apathy, decreased socialization, regression of motor control, and finally a comatose state have been reported in infants exclusively breastfed by vegan mothers. Although treatment with the vitamin generally brings complete reversal, at least one infant appeared not to have made full neurological recovery (27). Newborn infants normally have sufficient vitamin B-12 stores to support them through the first year, yet deficiencies of the vitamin have been seen at less than 6 months of age. Although maternal stores may protect the mother from deficiency, her stores are not readily available for placental transport to the developing fetus in amounts large enough to supply neonatal needs. Similarly, maternal stores are not readily available for secretion in breast milk because it is newly absorbed vitamin B-12 that can be utilized for cross-placental transport and secretion in the milk (28). The exclusively breastfed infant of a vegan mother whose vitamin B-12 intake is low may be predisposed to deficiency by a combination of low neonatal stores and low concentration in the breastmilk. It is imperative that all pregnant and lactating women, infants, and growing children be supplied with an adequate source of vitamin B-12.

Lactation places even greater energy demands on the mother than does pregnancy. Insufficient nutrient intake can affect the volume of milk produced. This may be of special importance for vegetarian infants who are usually breastfed for a prolonged time, often into the second year.

After 6 months of age, foods other than milk are needed for normal growth. Infants' and young children's stomachs are small, yet their energy and nutrient demands are great. Consequently, they need to consume foods of adequate density both as to energy and nutrients. Vegan and other restrictive diets may not supply enough calories per volume of food to support adequate growth. Shull et al. (22) suggested that some vegetarian infants may not receive supplemental weaning foods frequently enough or of a sufficiently high caloric density to support normal growth. These authors (22) found that vegetarian children, under age two, were smaller and growing more slowly than expected. Catch-up growth was only partially evident and not throughout the entire study population. Other studies have found anthropometric measurements of vegetarian children to be generally less than expected as compared to established standards, although vegetarian diets are not necessarily associated with leanness in children (23,29,30). How zinc and other nutriture relate to these findings are matters yet to be elucidated. Growth among LV and LOV children can be expected to approximate that of nonvegetarian children, while normal growth is harder to attain for children following more restricted diets (31). During periods of maximum growth the child is most vulnerable; however, it should be noted that optimal growth has yet to be rigorously defined.

Sanders and Purves (29) found energy intake in vegan children to be low in spite of their consumption of a large volume of food. Protein intake, assessed both quantitatively and qualitatively, was adequate for children whose parents were particularly knowledgeable in planning a vegetarian diet (29,30). Low calcium intake may impact on growth, especially when exacerbated by a low intake of vitamin D (29,30). Rickets has been documented among macrobiotic children (32). Homemade soymilk contains insufficient levels of necessary nutrients, and consumption of bovine milk or fortified soymilk should be encouraged.

Little research has been made into the nutritional status of teenage vegetarians. Hardinge and Stare (7) found no difference in height, weight, or various blood indices for adolescent vegetarians as compared to nonvegetarians. No recent studies have followed growth patterns of the "new" vegetarians through adolescence. Whether individuals are vegetarian or nonvegetarian, adolescent food habits may reflect a multitude of socio-psychological impacts. The understanding and well-informed parent can provide foods that will meet both the adolescent vegetarian's desires and nutrient needs.

Suggestions for dietary changes are more likely to be accepted if the philosophic constraints of the individual or family are kept in mind. Adequate nutritional support during pregnancy, use of appropriate supplemental weaning foods, intake of a wide variety of unrefined foods, and use of foods that are of sufficient caloric density to supply energy needs are all appropriate goals for any dietary lifestyle and should be encouraged among vegetarians as well as nonvegetarians.

Mineral and Vitamin Bioavailability

Nutritionists have raised questions about the lower bioavailability of trace minerals from a diet of unrefined cereals and legumes. These concerns are derived from the presence of phytate and the levels of dietary fiber. While refining improves the bioavailability of some trace minerals, it causes drastic loss of others (33). Sandstrom et al. (34), in their study of zinc absorption, showed that 38% of the zinc in white bread was absorbed as compared with only 17% of that in wholemeal bread. However, the absolute quantity of zinc absorbed from white bread was only two-thirds that absorbed from wholemeal bread. This occurred because wholemeal bread contains three times the zinc of the refined bread.

Phytate content has been of special concern in relation to zinc bioavailability. The leavening of wheat causes the phytate in bread to decrease by approximately 25%, thereby increasing zinc uptake by 30–50% (35). Hence, the leavening of wholemeal bread may result in an improved utilization of zinc. Sandstrom et al. (34) also showed that the addition of dairy products to wholemeal flour substantially increased the absorption of zinc. Lacto-vegetarians and LOVs typically consume considerable amounts of dairy products and ⅓ of their dietary zinc may come from this source. On the other hand, vegans, subsisting largely on fruits and vegetables, may have a low dietary zinc intake, thus resulting in an impaired zinc status (36).

Some concern has recently been expressed regarding the bioavailability of dietary iron and zinc in soybean-based foods. Short-term human studies show an impaired absorption of iron from soy protein as compared to meat protein (37). However, ascorbic acid is a potent facilitator of non-heme iron absorption. Vegetarians may consume increased quantities of this nutrient, thus facilitating their absorption of non-heme iron. Numerous vegetables, other foodstuffs, and beverages contain substantial quantities of organic acids (e.g., citric, malic, lactic, and tartaric acids), which also promote the absorption of non-heme iron (38). Animal and human absorption studies based on single test meals have shown that the bioavailability of zinc from soybean products is lower than that from animal products. Phytate, found largely in legumes, roots, and tubers, is known to complex with zinc to form an insoluble compound in the normal range of intestinal pH.

Long-term vegetarians have been reported as having adequate iron and zinc nutritional status. Zinc balance studies in college students in the Midwest revealed that the zinc in a vegetarian diet is better utilized by practicing vegetarians than by omnivores temporarily on a vegetarian diet. It appears that humans may adapt to the lower zinc bioavailability of vegetarian meals (39). However, Cossack and Prasad (40) recently found a compromised zinc status in male subjects who were fed a soy protein based diet for three months. They suggest that when soybean is the major protein source in a diet, dietary zinc of up to 15 mg per day may not be adequate to meet the adult human daily requirement. Nonetheless, biochemical indices of zinc nutriture have not conclusively identified long-term LOVs as being of poor zinc status. "New" vegetarians and vegans, however, may be at some risk of impaired zinc nutriture.

Certain vegetables contain oxalic acid, which can combine with calcium during digestion to form calcium oxalate, a compound that is not readily absorbed but is excreted in the feces (41). However, phytate and oxalic acid probably do not interfere with calcium absorption under normal dietary conditions wherein their concentrations are low relative to the amount of calcium present.

Although little is known about the effect of dietary fiber on the bioavailability of water- and fat-soluble vitamins, it has been reported that vitamins B-6 and B-12 may be unfavorably affected by high-fiber diets (42,43). These findings imply that the vitamin B-6 status of vegetarians may be lower than that of nonvegetarians—a matter of particular concern to the vegetarian female whose vitamin B-6 intake is below the RDA (15). In theory, having a low intake of vitamin B-12 could make a marginal vitamin B-12 status even more serious, due to the adverse effect of dietary fiber.

HEALTH AND DISEASE

Vegetarian diets offer the potential of decreasing the risk of onset of certain chronic degenerative diseases, such as obesity, high blood pressure, diabetes mellitus, coronary heart disease (CHD), colon and breast cancers, and osteoporosis (5).

Obesity

Obesity has been associated with a number of diseases (e.g., hypertension, CHD, diabetes mellitus, and endometrial and breast cancers). By the fifth decade, $1/3$ of American men and $1/2$ of the women are at least 20% overweight (5). Total vegetarians generally have body weights closer to the ideal than do nonvegetarians or LOVs (3,5). This could be related to high dietary fiber, low caloric density, or a greater emphasis on the control of intake by some TVs (5). Recent results from the Adventist Health Study reveal that nonvegetarian SDA men and women had a 50 to 100% greater prevalence of obesity (20% overweight or above) than did vegetarian SDA men and women (unpublished data). Some vegetarians are indeed obese; vegetarianism in and of itself may not protect against obesity.

Blood Pressure

Blood pressures (BPs) have been surveyed in societies throughout the world (44). Nonindustrialized societies tend to have lower levels than industrialized societies, blood pressures in the former showing little change with increasing age. Much emphasis has been placed upon the finding that groups which consume very little salt are at low risk both for hypertension and stroke. Nevertheless, there are some groups whose BP levels are quite low in spite of their consumption of moderate to high amounts of sodium (45,46). Studies have reported that vegetarians have lower BP levels than do nonvegetarians. No adequate explanation, however, has been given for these differences (47–49). Armstrong et al. (46) concluded that dietary sodium did not explain the blood pressure difference between vegetarians and nonvegetarians. So many variables distinguish vegetarian from nonvegetarian diets that it becomes important to identify which nutrients or factors may be the key regulators of blood pressure. Several studies have reported that a diet rich in polyunsaturated fatty acids tends to lower BP (50,51). Recently, Puska et al. (52) found that a diet low in fat and high in the ratio of polyunsaturated to saturated fatty acids significantly reduced BP, while sodium had little effect. The authors felt that this response was possibly induced through a change in the prostaglandin balance in both normotensives and hypertensives. We feel that a promising approach for prevention and nonpharmacological treatment of hypertension may lie in modifying one's dietary fat intake. However, it is premature to rule out the possible roles of other lifestyle and dietary factors.

Diabetes Mellitus

High-fiber diets containing approximately 60% of total calories as carbohydrates (75% of which are complex) tend to result in lower insulin requirements for diabetics than do corresponding low-fiber diets. Diabetic subjects who were taking nearly 30 units of insulin per day showed good blood glucose control without need of insulin after only a few weeks on a high complex carbohydrate diet (53). After six weeks on a high leguminous fiber diet, both insulin-dependent and non-insulin-dependent diabetics exhibited significantly lower fasting and postprandial blood glucose levels as well as lower total and low-density lipoprotein cholesterol levels (54).

The hypocholesterolemic effects of high-fiber diets in both normal and diabetic subjects result not only from a generous supply of water-soluble fiber but also from lower cholesterol and saturated fat contents and from a higher polyunsaturated-to-saturated fat ratio (55). A lower insulin requirement for diabetics on high-fiber diets would also translate into reduced hepatic cholesterol synthesis. Dietary fiber also binds bile salts and decreases their reabsorption. The interruption of the enterohepatic circulation of bile salts may be important to the hypocholesterolemic effect of dietary fiber.

Coronary Heart Disease

Certain subpopulations have unique lifestyles that make them fruitful groups to study in elucidating the roles of dietary factors in promoting or preventing disease. One such group are SDAs, members of a religious denomination that stresses healthful living. Aproximately 50% of SDAs consume an LOV diet, and almost all, even the nonvegetarians, refrain from eating pork products. These persons usually consume an abundant quantity of vegetables, fruits, whole grains, and nuts and generally abstain from the use of coffee, tea, alcoholic beverages, hot spicy condiments, and foods that are highly refined. For over 100 years, this type of dietary regimen has been strongly recommended for members of the church.

Phillips et al. (56) reported on CHD mortality rates in California SDAs as compared to the general population. They observed that male SDA vegetarians between the ages of 35 and 64 had a coronary heart disease mortality rate that was ⅓ that of male SDA nonvegetarians, suggesting that vegetarian diets may be associated with lower risk. The reduced saturated fat and cholesterol content of a vegetarian diet may not be the only factors in reducing risk. Lesser content of animal protein or high levels of complex carbohydrates may play important roles. The precise mechanism by which a group's lifestyle influences the risk of CHD is no doubt multiple in etiology and warrants further investigation.

Carroll (57) has reviewed the role of plant protein in lowering serum cholesterol and reducing the risk of atherosclerosis. These benefits are apart from the effects of fat composition or dietary cholesterol. The effect of protein on serum cholesterol may involve the amino acid composition of the diet. Kritchevsky et al. (58) suggest the lysine-to-arginine ratio as a predictor of atherogenesis in animals. Casein has a lysine-to-arginine ratio of 2.0 and is atherogenic, whereas soy protein has a lysine-to-arginine ratio of 1.0 and is antiatherogenic. Sirtori et al. (59) have shown that serum cholesterol levels were reduced in hypercholesterolemic subjects consuming soy protein diets. Sanchez et al. (60,61) recently found that several amino acids are altered as humans change from an omnivorous to a vegetarian diet. Plasma arginine was significantly increased in subjects fed a vegetarian diet for four weeks, while the lysine-to-arginine ratio was significantly decreased. Serum cholesterol also decreased significantly during the same period. The authors suggested that the amino acid content of dietary proteins may influence the level of plasma amino acids, which in turn may affect serum cholesterol and the atherogenic process. Furthermore, the hypocholesterolemic effect of soy protein diets may be mediated by increased fecal steroid excretion (62). Apart from the recognized value of polyunsaturated fats in reducing serum lipids and thrombosis, plant protein diets may be effective in the prevention and treatment of coronary atherosclerosis.

Polyunsaturated fats have been shown to inhibit thrombosis and prevent atherosclerosis (63). Diets containing substantial amounts of linoleic acid (the major polyunsaturated fatty acid in vegetable fats) cause a decrease in blood cholesterol levels, a decreased tendency toward thrombosis of platelets, and an improvement in heart function (64). Many of the actions of linoleic acid are mediated by the prostaglandins produced from linoleic acid metabolism; for example, adequate dietary linoleic acid decreases the synthesis of thromboxane A_2, a substance causing platelet aggregation. Linoleic acid levels have been found to be considerably lower in the serum phospholipids of heart attack patients than in those of normal subjects (65).

Cancer

In its review of potential dietary factors involved in the etiology of cancer, the Senate Select Committee on Nutrition and Human Needs suggested that Americans should increase their consumption of fruits, vegetables, and whole grains. This would imply an increase in consumption of dietary fiber. The interim dietary guidelines published by the Committee on Diet, Nutrition, and Cancer of the National Research Council likewise emphasized the importance of fruits, vegetables, and whole grains in the daily diet. Frequent consumption of these foods has been inversely associated with the incidence of various human cancers.

The mechanism by which dietary fiber protects against colon cancer is still poorly understood. Fiber decreases stool density and reduces transit time; thus carcinogens present in the stool may be diluted and have a briefer contact with the intestinal mucosa. Dietary fiber, together with fat intake, influences the type and metabolic activity of intestinal bacteria. Vegetarian populations are reported as having lower levels of anaerobic bacteria in the colon, thus possibly resulting in less carcinogenic secondary bile acids. Fiber components have also been shown to bind certain carcinogens, making them less available to act upon the intestinal mucosa. The anti-oxidant property of lignin may contribute to the ability of dietary fiber to protect against colon cancer.

Fruits and vegetables also contain other substances that are protective against cancer. A number of epidemiologic studies have shown that diets containing moderate to high levels of β-carotene are associated with a lesser risk of contracting lung and other cancers (66). Vitamin C interferes with the formation of carcinogenic nitrosamines. The cruciferous vegetables (e.g., cabbage, broccoli, cauliflower, and Brussels sprouts) contain indole compounds, which are known to stimulate the microsomal mixed function oxidase system that degrades chemical carcinogens (67). Graham et al. (68) have found that persons who consume cabbage at least once a week have one-third the risk of colon cancer relative to those who consume cabbage once a month or less.

The dietary hypothesis of cancer causation is further supported by the significant differences found in cancer mortality among populations existing in similar environs but possessing different dietary habits (69,70). In a study of food use in 37 countries, Drasar and Irving (71) showed that countrywide consumption of total fat, animal fat, and animal protein were all correlated with breast and colon cancer rates. Hill et al. (72) have shown in human feeding studies that the fat content of vegetarian and nonvegetarian regimens may affect the anterior pituitary or other glandular organs, thus modifying their response to the demands imposed by nutritional factors. Recently, Goldin et al. (73) and Shultz and Leklem (74) have shown that vegetarian and nonvegetarian diets may alter the metabolism of estrogen and prolactin in Caucasian pre-menopausal women. The latter findings of a positive association between estradiol-17β, estriol, and prolactin levels and dietary total fat, fatty acids, and protein tend further to support the hypothesis that specific dietary nutrients may modify hormonal balance and be of importance in human breast cancer etiology. Clearly, more research is needed in the identification of those dietary nutrients which may modify metabolic activity in a direction protective of the hormone dependent cancers.

Osteoporosis

Vegetarian women may be somewhat protected against the development of osteoporosis, a metabolic bone disease characterized by decreased bone mass and commonly affecting postmenopausal women. The high-protein diets typical of nonvegetarians are associated with an increased urinary excretion of calcium. The amino acids methionine and cysteine have been implicated in this altered kidney function (75). Animal proteins contain much higher levels of these sulfur-containing amino acids than do legumes. Marsh et al. (76) have shown that LOV women, aged 50–89 years, lost only 50% as much bone mineral mass when compared to omnivorous women. The higher sulfur content of the nonvegetarian diet was implicated in their findings, since both groups consumed similar levels of calcium (76).

DISCUSSION AND CONCLUSIONS

A vegetarian diet has been suggested as a practical means of reducing the risk of such chronic diseases as obesity, hypertension, diabetes mellitus, CHD, some cancers, and osteoporosis. Additionally, there is evidence that a vegetarian diet may serve as a treatment modality for some of these diseases. Different authors emphasize the value of different constituents of the vegetarian diet. There is little doubt that there are a number of nutritional factors which may play important roles in the prevention of certain diseases. The benefits of a vegetarian diet may be due, however, partly to the altered intake of various nutrients, partly to other substances in the food, and partly to various aspects of lifestyle which may be related to the choice of vegetarianism. Further research is certainly needed to clarify the mechanisms involved and to provide improved guidelines for the professional and a better understanding for the consumer.

It is often attractive for some advocates of a vegetarian diet to overemphasize its benefits. The LV or LOV diet can be nutritionally adequate for all persons, including infants, children, adolescents, pregnant women, and adults. The total vegetarian diet, when carefully planned, is also nutritionally adequate. A vegetarian diet, *per se*, is no reason for clinical or nutritional concern unless it is unusually restrictive as regards the quantity and variety of foods. Reliance on any single food source could lead to real nutritional risk. When vegetarian diets are well planned and skillfully implemented, no problems should arise regarding sufficient calories, adequate protein, and adequate levels of vitamins and minerals. Total vegetarians should pay special attention to the nutrients at risk and to the increased nutritional needs of pregnancy and periods of growth and development. Further study is needed to elucidate the long-term effects that restrictive vegetarian diets impose on infants' and children's physical and mental development.

Although only a small proportion of Americans are vegetarians (approximately 7 million), a growing number are accepting it as a practical dietary alternative. Many have changed their dietary preferences from the typical Western diet to some kind of vegetarianism. Many others do not consider themselves vegetarians but choose to limit their intake of animal foods. Many persons consuming a nonvegetarian diet perceive the change to a vegetarian diet as difficult and possibly hazardous. Such people need the assurance that no hazard exists provided the diet is balanced and well planned. Identical principles of sound menu planning apply to the vegetarian as to the nonvegetarian diet.

The well-known, four-food-group plan can be easily adapted for the LV or LOV, the major change being in substituting the protein-rich plant foods for meat and other animal foods. The following recommendations are important in using the four-food-group plan as a guide for devising an adequate vegetarian diet (2–5).

1. Decrease substantially the use of empty and highly-refined calories (e.g., sugar, jellies and jams, soft drinks, candies, most prepared desserts, refined breads and cereals, and visible fats). As far as possible, substitute unrefined foods that supply nutrients adequate to their calorie content.
2. Use vegetables and fruits freely, either raw or cooked, four or more servings per day. Use a daily variety that assures an adequate supply of vitamins A and C.
3. Increase the bread–cereal group beyond the recommended four servings if needed to meet energy requirements. Emphasize the use of whole grain breads and cereals; a variety of grain products should be used daily.
4. Provide two or more servings of non- or low-fat milk or dairy products. Servings from this group may be increased to supplement or substitute for the meat group.
5. Replace meat with an increased intake of plant proteins. Suitable plant protein sources include dried beans and peas, nuts, and meat analogs. Commercially prepared meat substitutes, although not essential to a well-balanced vegetarian diet, may help to make the transition easier from an omnivorous to a vegetarian diet. These convenience foods appease the palates of some persons and serve to replace meat entrees without requiring major changes in eating habits.

Planning a total vegetarian diet requires further considerations. The transition to a total vegetarian diet is made easier with the intermediate step of an LV or LOV diet. In addition to those for the LV or LOV diet, the following recommendations are important for a total vegetarian diet:

1. Maintain an adequate caloric intake by using breads, cereals, dried fruits, legumes, and nuts and seeds (e.g., sunflower and sesame seeds, soybeans).
2. Replace milk with foods that are good sources of the same nutrients found in milk. Since milk is an excellent source of calcium and riboflavin, the following recommendations should be followed:
   a. Use a fortified soybean milk.
   b. Increase the use of dark green leafy vegetables.
   c. Increase the use of legumes, especially soybeans, and nuts and seeds high in calcium.
   d. Use a modest amount of food yeast in meat analogs or other dishes.
3. Maintain an adequate protein supply by use of a variety of unrefined breads and cereals, legumes, and nuts and seeds.
4. Since there is no practical source of vitamins B-12 and D in plant foods, these vitamins must be furnished from other sources. Vitamin D can be supplied by sunlight on the skin. Vitamin B-12 can be supplied from B-12 fortified foods such as certain ready-to-eat cereals, soy milk, or meat analogs. If these are not used, supplements of vitamin B-12 should be taken.

Additional guidelines and practical considerations for pregnant and lactating women, infants, children, and adolescents have been previously mentioned. Finally, adoption of the basic nutrient principles of the U.S. Dietary Goals would help to prevent or delay the development of chronic degenerative diseases. These principles are generally met by well-balanced vegetarian diets (15), and include the following: (1) increasing the intake of complex carbohydrates so as to constitute some 55% of total calories (the intake of fats would then be reduced to 30% of total calories), (2) maintaining the intake of saturated fatty acids at approximately 10% of total calories, (3) replacing saturated fatty acids by mono- and polyunsaturates to a maximum of 10% of total caloric intake each, (4) limiting the intake of salt to about 5 g/day, (5) reducing cholesterol intake to less than 300 mg/day, and (6) adjusting caloric intake to achieve and maintain desirable weight. These recommendations are appropriate for the general population. The adoption of these modified dietary patterns at a sufficiently early age, if maintained for life, could result in long-term benefits to health and well-being.

REFERENCES

1. M. G. Hardinge and H. Crooks, Non-flesh dietaries, I. Historical background. *J. Am. Diet. Assoc.* **431**, 545 (1963).
2. The American Dietetic Association. *Handbook of Clinical Dietetics*, Yale University Press, New Haven, Conn., 1981.
3. L. Sonnenberg, K. Zolber, and U. D. Register, *Food For Us All, Revised Vegetarian Diet Study Kit*, The American Dietetic Association, Chicago, Ill, 1981.
4. M. K. Heath, *Diet Manual Including a Vegetarian Meal Plan*, 6th ed., The Seventh-Day Adventist Dietetic Association, Loma Linda, Cal., 1982.
5. J. J. B. Anderson, ed., *Nutrition and Vegetarianism*, Proceedings of Public Health Nutrition Update, Health Sciences Consortium, Chapel Hill, N.C., 1982.
6. U. D. Register and L. M. Sonnenberg, The vegetarian diet. Scientific and practical considerations. *J. Am. Diet. Assoc.* **62**, 253 (1973).
7. M. G. Hardinge and F. J. Stare, Nutritional studies of vegetarians, I. Nutritional, physical, and laboratory studies. *J. Clin. Nutr.* **2**, 73 (1954).
8. M. G. Hardinge and F. J. Stare, Nutritional studies of vegetarians, II. Dietary and serum levels of cholesterol. *J. Clin. Nutr.* **2**, 83 (1954).
9. P. T. Brown and J. G. Bergan, The dietary status of "new" vegetarians. *J. Am. Diet. Assoc.* **67**, 455 (1975).
10. M. H. Read and D. C. Thomas, Nutrient and food supplement practices of lacto-ovo vegetarians. *J. Am. Diet. Assoc.* **82**, 401 (1983).
11. S. P. Yang, J. E. Steinhauer, and J. O. Masterson, Utilization of a delayed lysine supplement by young rats. *J. Nutr.* **79**, 257 (1963).
12. A. Sanchez, J. A. Scharffenberg, and U. D. Register, Nutritive value of selected proteins and protein combinations. I. The biological value of proteins singly and in meal patterns with varying fat composition. *Am. J. Clin. Nutr.* **13**, 243 (1963).
13. A. Sanchez, G. G. Porter, and U. D. Register, Effect of entree on fat and protein quality of diets. *J. Am. Diet. Assoc.* **49**, 492 (1966).
14. M. G. Hardinge, H. Crooks, and F. J. Stare, Nutritional studies of vegetarians. V. Proteins and essential amino acids. *J. Am. Diet. Assoc.* **48**, 25 (1966).
15. T. D. Shultz and J. Leklem, Dietary status of Seventh-Day Adventists and nonvegetarians. *J. Am. Diet. Assoc.* **83**, 27 (1983).
16. E. R. Monsen, L. Hallberg, M. Layrisse, D. M. Hegsted, J. D. Cook, W. Mertz, and C. A. Finch, Estimation of available dietary iron. *Am. J. Clin. Nutr.* **31**, 134 (1978).
17. E. D. West and F. R. Ellis, The electroencephalogram in veganism, vegetarianism, vitamin B-12 deficiency and controls. *J. Neurol. Neurosurg. Psychiatry* **29**, 391 (1966).
18. F. R. Ellis and V. M. E. Montegriffo, Veganism, clinical findings and investigations. *Am. J. Clin. Nutr.* **23**, 249 (1970).

19. B. K. Armstrong, R. E. Davis, D. J. Nicol, A. J. Van Merwyk, and C. J. Larwood, Hematological, vitamin B-12, and folate studies on Seventh-Day Adventist vegetarians. *Am. J. Clin. Nutr.* **27**, 712 (1974).

20. T. A. B. Sanders, F. R. Ellis, and J. W. T. Dickerson, Hematological studies on vegans. *Br. J. Nutr.* **40**, 9 (1978).

21. J. Thomas, F. R. Ellis, and P. L. C. Diggory, The health of vegans during pregnancy. *Nutr. Soc. Proc.* **36**, 46A (1977), Abstract.

22. M. W. Shull, R. B. Reed, I. Valadian, R. Palombo, H. Thorne, and J. T. Dwyer, Velocities of growth in vegetarian preschool children. *Pediatrics* **60**, 410 (1977).

23. J. T. Dwyer, W. H. Dietz, E. M. Andrew, and R. M. Suskind, Nutritional status of vegetarian children. *Am. J. Clin. Nutr.* **35**, 204 (1982).

24. J. C. King, T. Stein, and M. Doyle, Effect of vegetarianism on the zinc status of pregnant women. *Am. J. Clin. Nutr.* **34**, 1049 (1981).

25. M. Abu-Assal and W. J. Craig, The zinc status of pregnant vegetarian women. *Nutr. Rep. Intl.* **29**, 485 (1984).

26. M. C. Higginbottom, L. Sweetman, and W. L. Nyhan, A syndrome of methylmalonic aciduria, homocystinuria, megaloblastic anemia and neurologic abnormalities in a vitamin B-12 deficient breast-fed infant of a strict vegetarian. *N. Engl. J. Med.* **299**, 317 (1978).

27. M. C. Wighton, J. I. Manson, I. Speed, E. Robertson, and E. Chapman, Brain damage in infancy and dietary vitamin B-12 deficiency. *Med. J. Australia* **2**, 1 (1979).

28. J. R. Davis, J. Goldenring, and B. H. Lubin, Nutritional vitamin B-12 deficiency in infants. *Am. J. Dis. Child.* **135**, 566 (1981).

29. T. A. B. Sanders and R. Purves, An anthropometric and dietary assessment of the nutritional status of vegan preschool children. *J. Hum. Nutr.* **35**, 349 (1981).

30. J. R. Fulton, C. W. Hutton, and K. R. Stitt, Preschool vegetarian children. *J. Am. Diet. Assoc.* **76**, 360 (1980).

31. W. C. MacLean and G. C. Graham, Vegetarianism in children. *Am. J. Dis. Child.* **134**, 513 (1980).

32. J. T. Dwyer, W. H. Dietz, G. Hass, and R. Suskind, Risk of nutritional rickets among vegetarian children. *Am. J. Dis. Child.* **133**, 134 (1979).

33. H. A. Schroeder, Losses of vitamins and trace minerals resulting from processing and preservation of foods. *Am. J. Clin. Nutr.* **24**, 562 (1971).

34. B. Sandstrom, B. Arvidsson, A. Cederblad, and E. Bjorn-Rasmussen, Zinc absorption from composite meals. I. The significance of wheat extraction rate, zinc, calcium, and protein content in meals based on bread. *Am. J. Clin. Nutr.* **33**, 739 (1980).

35. Zinc availability in leavened and unleavened bread. *Nutr. Rev.* **33**, 18 (1975).

36. J. H. Freeland-Graves, P. W. Bodzy, and M. A. Eppright, Zinc status of vegetarians. *J. Am. Diet. Assoc.* **77**, 655 (1980).

37. J. D. Cook, T. A. Morck, and S. R. Lynch, The inhibitory effect of soy products on nonheme iron absorption in man. *Am. J. Clin. Nutr.* **34**, 2622 (1981).
38. D. P. Derman, T. H. Bothwell, J. D. Torrance, W. R. Bezmoda, A. P. MacPhail, M. C. Kew, M. H. Sayers, P. B. Disler and R. W. Charlton, Iron absorption from maize (Zea mays) and sorghum (Sorghum vulgare) beer. *Br. J. Nutr.* **43**, 271 (1980).
39. C. Kies, E. Young, and L. McEndree, Zinc bioavailability from vegetarian diets. In G. E. Inglett, ed., *Nutritional Bioavailability of Zinc*, American Chemical Society, Washington, D.C., 1983, p. 115.
40. Z. T. Cossack and A. S. Prasad, Effect of protein source on the bioavailability of zinc in human subjects. *Nutr. Res.* **3**, 23 (1983).
41. U. Pingle, and B. V. Ramasastri, Absorption of calcium from a leafy vegetable rich in oxalates. *Br. J. Nutr.* **39**, 119 (1978).
42. J. Leklem, L. T. Miller, A. D. Perera, and D. E. Pfeffers, Bioavailability of vitamin B-6 from wheat bread in humans. *J. Nutr.* **110**, 1819 (1980).
43. R. W. Cullen and S. M. Oace, Methylmalonic acid and vitamin B-12 excretion of rats consuming diets varying in cellulose and pectin. *J. Nutr.* **108**, 640 (1978).
44. F. H. Epstein and R. D. Eckoff, The epidemiology of high blood pressure: Geographic distributions and etiological factors. In J. Stamler, R. Stamler, and R. Pullman, eds., *The Epidemiology of Hypertension*, Grune and Stratton, New York, 1967, p. 155.
45. T. Kimura and M. Ota, Epidemiologic study of hypertension: Comparative results of hypertensive surveys in two areas in Northern Japan. *Am. J. Clin. Nutr.* **17**, 381 (1965).
46. B. Armstrong, H. Clarke, C. Martin, W. Ward, N. Norman, and J. Masarei, Urinary sodium and blood pressure in vegetarians. *Am. J. Clin. Nutr.* **32**, 2472 (1979).
47. F. M. Sacks, B. Rosner, and E. H. Kass, Blood pressure in vegetarians. *Am. J. Epidemiol.* **100**, 390 (1974).
48. B. Armstrong, A. J. Van Merwyk, and H. Coates, Blood pressure in Seventh-Day Adventist vegetarians. *Am. J. Epidemiol.* **105**, 444 (1977).
49. A. C. Anholm, The relationship of a vegetarian diet to blood pressure. *Prev. Med.* **7**, 35 (1978).
50. J. M. Iacono, M. W. Marshall, R. M. Dougherty, M. A. Wheeler, J. F. Markin, and J. J. Canary, Reduction in blood pressure associated with high polyunsaturated fat diets that reduce blood cholesterol in man. *Prev. Med.* **4**, 426 (1975).
51. B. Stern, S. Heyden, D. Miller, G. Latham, A. Klimas, and K. Pilkington, Intervention study in high-school students with elevated blood pressures: Dietary experiment with polyunsaturated fatty acids. *Nutr. Metab.* **24**, 137 (1980).
52. P. Puska, A. Nissinen, E. Vartiainen, R. Dougherty, M. Mutanen, J. M. Iacono, H. J. Korhonen, P. Pietinen, U. Leino, S. Moisio, and J.

Huttunen, Controlled, randomised trial of the effect of dietary fat on blood pressure. *Lancet* 1, 3 (1983).

53. J.W. Anderson, High-fiber diets for diabetic and hypertriglyceridemic patients. *Can. Med. Assoc. J.* 123, 975 (1980).

54. H.C.R. Simpson, A high leguminous fibre diet improves all aspects of diabetic control. *Lancet* 1, 1 (1981).

55. R.M. Kay and A.S. Truswell, Dietary fiber: Effects on plasma and biliary lipids in man. In G.A. Spiller and R.M. Kay, eds., *Medical Aspects of Dietary Fiber*, Plenum, New York, 1980, p. 153.

56. R.L. Phillips, R.F. Lemon, W.L. Beeson, and J.W. Kuzma, Coronary heart disease mortality among Seventh-Day Adventists with differing dietary habits: A preliminary report. *Am. J. Clin. Nutr.* 31, S191 (1978).

57. K.K. Carroll, Hypercholesterolemia and atherosclerosis: Effects of dietary protein. *Fed. Proc.* 41, 2792 (1982).

58. D. Kritchevsky, S.A. Tepper, S.K. Czarnecki, and D.M. Klurfeld, Atherogenicity of animal and vegetable protein—Influence of the lysine to arginine ratio. *Atherosclerosis* 41, 429 (1982).

59. C.R. Sirtori, E. Gatti, O. Mantero, R. Conti, E. Agradi, E. Tremoli, M. Sirtori, L. Fraterrigo, L. Tavassi, and D. Kritchevsky, Clinical experience with the soybean-protein diet in treatment of hypercholesterolemia. *Am. J. Clin. Nutr.* 32, 1645 (1979).

60. A. Sanchez, M.C. Horning, and D.C. Wengelith, Plasma amino acids in humans fed plant protein. *Nutr. Rep. Intl.* 28, 497 (1983).

61. A. Sanchez, M.C. Horning, J. Harris, G. Shavlik, and D.C. Wengelith, Plasma amino acids associated with hypercholesterolemia, Western Hemisphere Nutrition Congress VII, Miami Beach, Fla. (1983), Abstract.

62. J.A. Story and D. Kritchevsky, Influence of dietary protein on cholesterol metabolism. *J. Am. Oil Chem. Soc.* 60, 696 (1983), Abstract.

63. A.J. Vergroesen, Physiological effects of dietary linoleic acid. *Nutr. Rev.* 35, 1 (1977).

64. S.H. Goodnight, W.S. Harris, W.E. Connor, and D.R. Illingworth. Polyunsaturated fatty acids, hyperlipidemia, and thrombosis. *Arteriosclerosis* 2, 87 (1982).

65. T.A. Miettinen, V. Naukkarinen, J.K. Huttunen, S. Mattila, and J. Kumlin, Fatty acid composition of serum lipids predicts myocardial infarction. *Br. Med. J.* 285, 993 (1982).

66. G. Wolf, Is dietary β-carotene an anti-cancer agent? *Nutr. Rev.* 40, 257 (1982).

67. L.W. Wattenberg, Effects of dietary constituents on the metabolism of chemical carcinogens. *Cancer Res.* 35, 3326 (1975).

68. S. Graham, H. Dayal, M. Swanson, A. Mittelman, and G. Wilkinson, Diet in the epidemiology of cancer of the colon and rectum. *J. Natl. Cancer Inst.* 61, 709 (1978).

69. R.L. Phillips, Role of life-style and dietary habits in risk of cancer among Seventh-Day Adventists. *Cancer Res.* 35, 3513 (1975).

70. J.E. Enstrom, Cancer mortality among Mormons. *Cancer* 36, 825 (1975).

71. B. S. Drasar and D. Irving, Environmental factors and cancer of the colon and breast. *Br. J. Cancer* **27**, 167 (1973).

72. P. Hill, L. Garbaczewski, P. Helman, J. Huskisson, E. Sporangisa, and E. L. Wynder. Diet, lifestyle, and menstrual activity. *Am. J. Clin. Nutr.* **33**, 1192 (1980).

73. B. R. Goldin, H. Adlercreutz, S. L. Gorbach, J. H. Warram, J. T. Dwyer, L. Swenson, and M. N. Woods, Estrogen excretion patterns and plasma levels in vegetarian and omnivorous women. *New Engl. J. Med.* **307**, 1542 (1982).

74. T. D. Shultz and J. E. Leklem, Comparative nutrient intake and hormonal interrelationships among healthy premenopausal vegetarian Seventh-Day Adventists, and non-vegetarians. *Nutr. and Cancer* **4**, 247 (1983).

75. H. M. Linkswiler, M. B. Zemel, M. Hegsted, and S. Schuette, Protein-induced hypercalciuria. *Fed. Proc.* **40**, 2429 (1981).

76. A. G. Marsh, T. V. Sanchez, O. Michelsen, J. Keiser, and G. Mayor, Cortical bone density of adult lacto-ovo-vegetarian and omnivorous women. *J. Am. Diet. Assoc.* **76**, 148 (1980).

8
Wild Foods for Modern Diets

HARRIET V. KUHNLEIN, Ph.D., R.D.
Division of Human Nutrition
University of British Columbia
Vancouver, Canada

Address correspondence to Harriet V. Kuhnlein, Ph.D., Associate Professor of Nutrition, Division of Human Nutrition, University of British Columbia, Vancouver, British Columbia, Canada V6T 1W5.

ABSTRACT

There are thousands of wild plant and animal species in the world today that could contribute meaningfully to human nutrition. These foods would be especially beneficial to persons with low income and to those living in areas where there is limited availability and variety in marketed foods. They can also be used to enhance genetically existing agricultural crops, and to develop new crops for commercial distribution. More documentation is needed on wild foods for: (1) use and preparation by indigenous people, (2) environmental availability and growth requirements, (3) acceptability by contemporary consumers, (4) toxicological properties, and (5) nutrient composition. This chapter discusses the use of wild foods and where published information can be obtained about them. Emphasis is given to the potential nutritional contributions they might make to modern diets. The chapter concludes with some general principles for counseling individuals who wish to use wild foods available in their area.

WHAT ARE WILD FOODS?

Wild foods can be defined as species of noncultivated plants, fish, game, and other animal life that have been used as foods by indigenous, native, or Indian people. These foods are usually not subjected to systematic farming, be it commercial agriculture or home or community gardening or husbandry. In the distant past, before the beginnings of agriculture, all of mankind was nourished by wild species of foods. The "Neolithic Revolution," which commonly denotes that period when the majority of humans made the transition from hunter–gatherers to an agricultural society, occurred within the last 1% of the two million or so years that cultural man has been on earth. The reasons for this prehistoric adaptation to agriculture have been considered in detail elsewhere (1,2) and will not be discussed here. Suffice it to say that all of our contemporary plant and animal agricultural crops have their origins in wild species (3). The reasons why some wild species were selected over other wild contemporaries for

154

agricultural development remains obscured in history, but it is clear that there are thousands of little known and underutilized foods in their unique ecological niches of the world today. Iker (4) estimates that of a possible 80,000 edible plants in the world, only about 3000 species have been exploited over the course of history. Currently, a major share of the world's human food energy is harvested in the massive agriculture of just three cereals—wheat, rice, and corn (4).

With the everpresent concerns for environmental damage by industrialized civilization, it is time to document our wild foods, to study their nutritional and esthetic properties, and to develop them to their full potential for meeting human food needs. This review describes how wild foods can be utilized, and identifies sources of literature on the use and nutrient composition of North American wild foods.

POTENTIAL USES OF WILD FOODS

If we accept Iker's estimation that there are more than 70,000 species of underutilized edible plants in the world and add to this a similar magnitude of edible animal species, the possibilities for additional foods in our diets are staggering. What would be the benefits of developing the informational base and use of wild plant and animal foods?

Source of Food and Nutrients in Low-Income Diets

Because wild foods, by definition, do not enter the agricultural complex, they are usually not marketed. Although monetary value is not at issue for these foods, the actual time and labor costs may be considerable for harvesting and preparation, as well as preservation. Rural residents will usually have greater access to most wild foods on a yearly basis, although some wild plant species are readily available in the vacant lots and alleyways of urban areas (5). Because of the need for transportation to rural areas, it may be more "costly" for urban residents to access a spectrum of wild foods from rural areas.

If public knowledge of these foods is made available, and the foods can be reasonably accessed, significant contributions to family meals can be made. Many low-income people in the Canadian north depend on large game animals (venison, moose) for winter meat supplies. Berries, edible leafy plants, and fish can also provide a large proportion of needed vitamins and minerals. In remote areas where marketed foods are limited in variety, these foods can be exceptionally useful as nutrient supplements. Their usefulness can be extended into other seasons with the common methods of home food preservation: canning, freezing, and drying.

The ecological density of wild food resources should be carefully considered before extensive harvesting is undertaken. While some species may be plentifully abundant (consider dandelions, for example), others may be jeopardized with extinction if overharvested. Two Lileaceous root foods of native people in the Pacific Northwest, camas (*Camassia* spp.) and riceroot (*Fritillaria* spp.), have been seriously depleted by the overgrazing of domestic animals and habitat destruction following industrialization. Overharvesting of these plants could now threaten them with extinction (6).

Revival of Cultural Food Patterns of Native People

Although the milieu of commercial foods has displaced the native diet in many parts of the world (7,8), there has been an effort by many native groups to document their cultural foods and to revive their use as much as is possible. This has occurred primarily among people who have retained lands they occupied before "white" contact, and who still have an older generation who can recall the traditional, often "wild" foods. Such groups are eager for scientific documentation on the nutritional properties of their foods, since it is strongly felt that the traditional diet would improve health conditions as well as the cultural morale in native communities. In addition, traditional Indian foods are promoted as low-cost sources of nutrients in areas where purchasing power may be limited because of reduced income or lack of food markets.

Some of the most popular and available native traditional foods have been retained over the years by native people who continue to live in their original environment. Examples of these are the use of rendered fish oil by Northwest people, wild desert greens by the Hopi and Papago of Arizona, and the use of soapberries to make "Indian ice cream" by most Indian groups living in coastal or interior regions of British Columbia (9–12).

Development of "New" Foods

Many people are eager to explore the new tastes and textures that these foods offer. For these individuals, the foods need only to be brought to their attention and made available. The well-known popularity of wild strawberries, raspberries, lingonberries, mushrooms, and game meats in Europe is good evidence of this. European food entrepreneurs have even attempted to import unusual plant foods used by native North Americans for marketing to higher income families wishing new cultural food adventures (Jurgen Boden, Leine, W. Germany, personal communication). Another example is the demand for wild green plant foods in the commercial markets of urban Mexico. Several of these plants have been documented recently (13).

The continuing attention received by the "health food movement" (from a variety of personal perspectives) also contributes to the acceptance of wild foods by the general public. Many are convinced to incorporate into family meals more foods which are "unrefined, unprocessed, and natural." The appeal of wild foods to this audience is obvious. Unfortunately, health food stores are known to capitalize by exaggerating the nutritional properties of some wild foods (rosehips, honey, seaweed, etc.) when actual analyses on their dietary contributions may not have been done.

Despite these problems, use of several wild foods from the near environment could make a pleasant contribution to variety in family meals. This is especially true in remote areas where the extent of marketed foods is limited, or where low income limits purchasing. As mentioned, however, wild foods are also attractive to families with greater purchasing power.

Many wild plants, such as sheep sorrel (*Rumex* spp.) or purslane (*Portullaca* spp.), can be simply planted and harvested. Genetic stocks of other species can be used to create new agricultural crops or to enhance existing crops. To this end, germplasm conservation programs and wild food data banks are valuable resources (14,15). The astonishing agricultural success of the winged bean (*Psophocarpus tetragonolobus*), a tropical legume from Southeast Asia, for food production in many developing areas of the world is well documented (16). Another example of a wild plant improving the genetic stock of a domesticated crop is the use of the Mexican teosinte maize with commercial varieties (17).

There is a great potential for many native food plants to enhance genetically existing crops and for the horticultural development of new foods for cultivation and marketing. Within North America, several commercially grown fruits have been derived or improved with wild species: strawberry, blackberry, gooseberry, American cranberry, and blueberry, among others. Wild rice, Jerusalem artichokes, maple syrup, black walnuts, pecans, pinyon nuts, and chia seeds are some other North American wild food plants that are in common use and are found in North American markets (18,19). The possibilities for new foods to be readily received in markets is considerable in some areas. Mexican migrant laborers in Tucson have created a market for *Amaranthus* spp., *Chenopodium* spp., and *Portulaca* spp., all wild, leafy green plants native **to desert regions (Dr. Gary Nabhan, Arid Lands Studies, Tucson,**

Arizona, personal communication). These are harvested from wild plots and sold in roadside stands or open markets.

The possibilities for propagating, even cultivating, wild plant species for personal consumption needs further study. Programs such as Native Seeds/SEARCH (3950 W. New York Drive, Tucson, Arizona, 85745) will help to ensure that indigenous plant foods known and used by native people will not be overharvested and threatened with extinction. Hopefully, many species of wild plants and animals can be intelligently managed to take their place in the diets of all those who wish them.

It is clear that wild foods hold much promise for enhancing our food supplies. There is a pressing need for investigating these resources and documenting their nutritional properties, palatability and overall acceptability, availability, methods of harvest and preparation used by native people, and their potential toxicology.

Wilderness Survival and Environmental Education

Knowledge about the occurrence and use of wild foods has been avidly used by instructors of courses in wilderness survival. Camp counselors, "Outward-bound" leaders, wilderness guides, even the military establishment, have been gathering knowledge on the use of wild foods for the training of people who will be living in remote areas. For these people, knowledge on availability, preparation, nutrient contents, and possible toxicology of these foods is essential information.

General education programs that emphasize environmental awareness also give information and encouragement to use wild food resources. These programs teach the ecological conditions needed for the growth of wild species, and how environmental deterioration has contributed to the reduced availability, especially of game animals. Some curricula also present the potential nutritional contributions to humans that these foods offer.

WHERE TO FIND INFORMATION ON WILD FOODS

The best place to find background information on edible species of wild foods for a given area is to search the ethnographic literature. Documentation of the subsistence strategies of native people can be found in the reports of archeologists, anthropologists, and ethnobiologists who worked in the region. These should be available in public libraries, government archives, and university libraries, as well as in ethnographic museums. These ethnographic accounts might provide insights on seasonal use, methods of harvest and preparation, as well as general appeal.

Other sources give descriptive information on how to identify and use edible wild plants, and can be broad or regional in scope. Examples of these are: Sturtevant's *Edible Plants of the World* (20) by E. L. Sturtevant, *Edible and Useful Wild Plants of the United States and Canada* (21) by C. F. Saunders, *Edible Wild Plants of the Great Lakes Region* (22) by Weatherbee and Bruce, and *Guide to Common Edible Plants of British Columbia* (23) by Szczawinski and Hardy. Similar composites of information for wild animal foods are more difficult to find, but are also more generalizable. Extension pamphlets such as Burand's *Alaska's Game is Good Food* (24) provide information on venison, caribou, reindeer, moose, buffalo, muskrat, bear, beaver, whale, walrus, and squirrel. In addition, most comprehensive cook books, such as those by Montagne (25), Ellis and Simpkins (26), and Rombauer and Becker (27), give methods of preparation of game.

Information on toxicological properties and nutrient composition of wild foods is usually more difficult to find. General toxicological references such as the National Academy of Sciences publication *Toxicants Occurring Naturally in Foods* (28) and *Poisonous Plants of the United States and Canada* (29) by Kingsbury can be broadly informative. The series of four publications by Turner and Szczawinski (two of these by Szczawinski and Turner) responsibly give warnings on the potentially toxic effects of consuming certain wild foods indiscriminately (5,30−32). These authors make it very clear to the lay reader that wild plant foods must be carefully identified and prepared. However, for the majority of edible wild plants of North America, systematic toxicological evaluations have not been made. This being the case, edibility and safety of species must be inferred from patterns of food use by indigenous peoples.

Information on the nutritional composition of wild species of plant and animal foods is very incomplete when compared to that available for marketed foods. Data on some wild species is given in the world's major tables of food composition, especially those volumes published by the United Nations' Food and Agriculture Organization (33−36). Other references containing some wild food data for North America are Watt and Merrill (37) and the recent major revision documents, as well as Pennington and Church (38), and the Canadian data table published by National Health and Welfare (39). The annotated bibliography compiled by Robson and Elias (40) is a good source of references containing original research data on many indigenous North American plants.

Table 1 is presented to assist the reader in locating major sources of nutrient information on wild North American foods. These are

Table 1. Selected Published Works Containing Numerous Nutrient Values for North American Wild Foods

Foods	Geographic Area	References	Numbe
Plant foods			
Indian food plants	North America	Yanovsky and Kingsbury (1938)	41
Indian foods	Eastern Canada	Arnason et al. (1981)	42
Indian foods	Arizona	Calloway et al. (1974)	43
Hopi Indian foods	Arizona	Kuhnlein et al. (1979)	11
Warm Springs Indian foods	Oregon	Benson et al. (1973)	44
Northwest Indian foods	Washington and Northern Oregon	Keely (1980)	45
Papago Indian foods	Arizona	Meals for Millions (1980)	10
Leaf foods	Tropics	Martin and Ruberte (1975)	46
Forest fruits and nuts	Pennsylvania	Wainio and Forbes (1941)	47
Wildlife foods	Connecticut	Spinner and Bishop (1950)	48
Food plants	U.S. and Canada	Beeson et al. (1971)	49
Arctic plant foods	Arctic	Brown (1954)	50
Wild plants	Ohio and Kentucky	Zennie and Ogzewalla (1977)	51
Alpine foods	North American alpine tundra	Johnston et al. (1968)	52
Wild plants	Alaska	Drury and Smith (1953)	53
Wild foods	North America	King and McClure (1944)	54
Alaskan foods	Alaska	Mann et al. (1962)	55
Marine algae	Nova Scotia	MacPherson (1949)	56
Vegetable foods	Cuba	Navia et al. (1955a) (1957);	57, 58
		Lopez et al. (1963)	59
Animal foods			
Indian meat and fish	Canada	Farmer and Neilson (1967) (1970);	60, 61
		Farmer et al. (1978)	62
Marine mammals	Northern Canada	Hoppner et al. (1978)	63
Animal foods	Arctic and Subarctic	Speth and Spielman (1983)	64
Insects	Mexico	Ramos Elorduy de Conconi (1982)	65
General references			
Many foods	North America	Watt and Merrill (1975)	37
Many foods	North America	Pennington and Church (1980)	38
Many foods	Latin America	Leung and Flores (1961)	36
Many foods	Canada	National Health and Welfare (1979)	39
Many foods	Caribbean	Caribbean Food and Nutrition Inst. (1974)	66
Many foods	Hawaii	Murai et al. (1958)	67

Table 2. Nutrient Composition of Commercial and Wild Northwest Berries[a]

Common Name/Botanical Name	CHO (g/100g)	Protein (g/100g)	Fat (g/100g)	Ca (mg/100g)	Fe (mg/100g)	Vitamin C (mg/100g)	Vitamin A (I.U./100g)	References
Commercial								
Strawberries/ *Fragaria virginiana*	8.4	0.7	0.5	21.0	1.0	59.0	60	37,39
Raspberries/ *Rubus idaeus*	13.8	1.2	0.5	22.0	0.9	25.0	130	37,39
Blueberries/ *Vaccinium myrtilloides*	15.3	0.7	0.5	15.0	1.0	14.0	100	37,39
Blackberries/ *Rubus allegheniensis*	12.9	1.2	0.9	32.0	0.9	21.0	200	37,39
Gooseberries/ *Ribes divaricatum*	9.7	0.8	0.2	18.0	0.5	33.0	290	37,39
Mean[b]	12.0	0.9	0.5	21.6	0.9	30.0	156	
Wild								
Thimbleberries/ *Rubus parviflorus*	24.7	3.1	1.2	129.2	0.9	78.0	—[c]	45
Salmonberries/ *Rubus spectabilis*	11.2	1.1	0.3	20.3	1.2	30.4	787	45,55[d]
Soapberries/ *Shepherdia canadensis*	—	2.3	0.3	20.0	—	—	—	12[d]
Salal berries/ *Gaultheria shallon*	14.0	2.1	0.7	51.6	0.7	68.5	—	45
Blackcaps/ *Rubus leucodermis*	15.7	1.5	—	30.0	1.1	48.7	—	68
Mean[b]	16.4	2.0	0.6	50.2	0.9	48.7	—	—

[a] All raw.

[b] Mean computed from known values.

[c] Not determined.

[d] Includes unpublished data from Kuhnlein (1980), Hooper (1981), and Pietarinen (1979).

published works that are prime sources of numerous nutrient values for North American wild plant and animal foods. There are innumerable published references that give less extensive information on a few foods, but these data are still being compiled.

NUTRIENT COMPOSITION OF WILD FOODS

In general, it can be assumed that if a wild food species is available, palatable, and devoid of toxic constituents, the nutrient profile can be expected to be at least as good as a marketed food in kind. In fact,

Table 3. Nutrient Composition of Commercial and Wild Root Foods [a]

Common Name/Botanical Name	CHO (g/100g)	Protein (g/100g)	Ca (mg/100g)	P (mg/100g)	Mg (mg/100g)	Fe (mg/100g)	Zn (mg/100g)	References
Commercial								
Potato (with skin) /*Solanum tuberosum*	17.1	2.1	9.3	39.4	22.0	0.5	0.2	38,69
Carrots/*Daucus carota*	9.7	1.1	37.0	36.0	18.0	0.7	0.5	70
Sweet potato/*Ipomoea batatas*	26.3	1.7	32.0	47.0	31.0	0.7	—[c]	38
Parsnips/*Pastinaca sativa*	17.5	1.7	50.0	77.0	32.0	0.7	—	38
Mean[b]	**17.7**	**1.7**	**32.1**	**49.8**	**26.0**	**0.7**	**0.4**	
Wild								
Clover/*Trifolium wormskioldii*	13.2	1.8	38.4	25.8	38.6	4.6	0.2	69
Silverweed/*Potentilla pacifica*	19.5	1.6	41.0	52.9	49.1	9.1	0.5	69
Camas/*Camassia quamash*	23.0	3.4	104.0	270.0	52.0	9.9	2.7	6,45
Wapato/*Sagittaria latifolia*	21.2	4.7	11.5	165.0	15.9	6.6	0.7	45,71
Mean[b]	**19.2**	**2.9**	**39.9**	**128.0**	**38.9**	**7.6**	**1.0**	

[a] All samples were raw. [b] Mean computed from known values only. [c] Not determined.

close investigation of nutrient contents of wild foods can reveal surprisingly high contents of some nutrients. To illustrate this, Tables 2, 3, and 4 give the composition of seven nutrients in several species of universally known commercial plant foods and a comparable number of wild plant foods found in North America. In Table 2, five berries typically found in North American markets are listed with five species of Northwest berries. The values for carbohydrate (CHO), protein, and fat are reasonably similar, but the wild berries tend to have more calcium, iron, and vitamin C. Vitamin A content (carotene) is shown for only one wild berry, the salmonberry, but it greatly exceeds that found in the commercial varieties. Thimbleberries (*Rubus parviflorus*) and salal berries (*Gaultheria shallon*) are excellent sources of calcium and vitamin C, in comparison to the commercial species.

Nutrients in four species of wild root foods are compared to common commercial species in Table 3. Carbohydrate and protein contents of the wild foods, in comparison to the commercial species, are again

Table 4. Nutrient Composition of Commercial and Wild Southwest Green Vegetables

Common Name/Botanical Name (Preparation)	Protein (g/100g)	Ca (mg/100g)	Fe (mg/100g)	Mg (mg/100g)	Zn (mg/100g)	Vitamin C (mg/100g)	Vitamin A (I.U./100g)	References
Commercial								
Iceberg lettuce/ *Lactuca sativa* (raw)	0.9	20.0	0.5	11.0	0.1	6.0	330	70
Spinach/ *spinacea oleracea* (boiled)	3.0	113.0	2.1	42.0	0.5	19.0	7900	70
Celery/ *Apium graveolens* (raw)	0.9	39.0	0.3	22.0	—[b]	9.0	240	70
Peas/ *Pisum sativum* (frozen, boiled)	5.1	19.0	1.9	21.0	0.9	13.0	600	70
Mean[a]	2.5	48.0	1.2	24.7	0.5	12.0	2268	
Wild								
Goosefoot/ *Chenopodium fremontii* (raw)	2.1	258.0	1.2	—	—	80.0	11600	10,36
Purslane/ *Portulaca oleraceae* (raw)	1.7	119.5	4.2	560.0	0.3	26.2	869	36,51,72
Amaranth/ *Amaranthus retroflexus* (boiled)	4.2	323.0	6.8	150.4	0.6	56.5	2333	73–75,36
Beeweed/ *Cleome serulata* (boiled)	8.1	209.0	2.1	32.0	1.0	—	—	c
Mean[a]	4.0	227.4	3.6	247.0	0.6	54.2	4934	

[a] Mean computed from known values only. [b] Not determined. [c] Unpublished data of Weber, et al. (1983).

similar. Although the mean calcium values are close, the contents for camas (*Camassia quamash*) exceed all other roots in the table. Camas is also high in phosphorus, as is wapato (*Sagittaria latifolia*). All of the wild species are quite high in iron (4.6–9.9 mg/100 g) in comparison to the more usually consumed vegetables (0.5–0.7 mg/100 g). Zinc is also unusually high in the camas.

In Table 4, two species of raw vegetables and two species of cooked vegetables are presented in the commercial and wild categories. Iceberg lettuce, spinach, celery, and peas are compared with goosefoot (*Chenopodium fremontii*), purslane (*Portulaca oleraceae*), amaranth (*Amaranthus retroflexus*), and beeweed (*Cleome serulata*). All species of the wild vegetables are shown to be higher in calcium than are any commercial species, and two of the four wild species are higher in iron and magnesium. The three wild species for which ascorbate data are available also demonstrate that the wild species have superior contents for this vitamin (mean of 54.2 versus 12.0 mg/100g). Carotene (vitamin A) in the leafy green plants is known to be high, and this is borne out in the data for spinach, goosefoot, and amaranth.

It is true that reported values for the commercial varieties are mean values from cross-national sampling, whereas values for the wild samples are probably taken from fewer samples in limited geographic location. Nevertheless, the high nutrient contents of these regionally available wild foods cannot be discounted, and their contributions to the dietary intake of individuals in their geographic areas could be considerable.

A series of commercially refined and indigenous salts have been compared for trace element contents and reported in 1980 (76). It was found that the indigenous salts contained the highest levels of all trace elements in contrast to the commercial salts. Salts of plant origin were the richest source of trace elements.

CONCLUSIONS

There are many species of wild plant and animal foods that are not fully utilized, and which could make meaningful contributions to modern diets in most parts of the world. For better utilization of our wild foods, we must increase our knowledge of their specific growth conditions and availability, their acceptability to consumers, and their composition for potential toxins and nutrients. Use of wild foods is especially relevant to individuals with low income and/or who are living in remote areas where marketed foods are limited in variety. They can also be developed to provide new and unusual foods for commercial markets.

When counseling individuals who wish to make use of wild foods in their area, the following principles should be emphasized:

1. Only harvest those species that are well known as human foods. Consult the ethnographies of the area, and be certain you can identify the correct species. This may require a training session by a biologist (botanist or wildlife specialist) familiar with your area. If you are in doubt about the possible toxicity of a species, get a positive identification before eating it.
2. Consider the time, energy, and other resources needed to harvest and prepare wild foods. Are these offset by the cultural, esthetic, and nutritional benefits that these foods will provide?

3. Develop an understanding of the ecology of the area, and do not overharvest any species. Be familiar with the propagation of plant species, and leave enough to replenish supplies for the next harvest season.

At this time, we need to expand the scientific knowledge base on wild species of plant and animal foods, so that the best use can be made of all of our food resources.

ACKNOWLEDGMENTS

The author expresses appreciation and thanks for review of the manuscript to Dr. Nancy Turner and Dr. Richard Ford. Mrs. Sandra Marquis and Mrs. Joanne Condruk assisted with manuscript preparation, and are also sincerely acknowledged.

REFERENCES

1. R. B. Lee and I. DeVore, eds., *Man the Hunter.* Aldine, Chicago, 1968.
2. M. N. Cohen, *The Food Crisis in Prehistory.* Yale University Press, New Haven, 1977.
3. P. J. Ucko and G. W. Dimbleby, eds., *The Domestication and Exploitation of Plants and Animals.* Aldine, Chicago, 1967.
4. S. Iker, Are you ready for the new foods? *Int. Wildlife* **9**, 28 (1979).
5. A. F. Szczawinski and N. J. Turner, *Edible Garden Weeds of Canada.* National Museum of Natural Sciences, Ottawa, 1978.
6. N. J. Turner and H. V. Kuhnlein, Camas (*Camassia* spp.) and riceroot (*Fritillaria* spp.): two Liliaceous "root" foods of the northwest coast Indians. *Ecol. Food and Nutr.* **13**, 199 (1983).
7. J. R. K. Robson, Commentary: Changing food habits in developing countries. *Ecol. Food Nutr.* **4**, 251 (1976).
8. H. V. Kuhnlein and D. H. Calloway, Contemporary Hopi food intake patterns. *Ecol. Food Nutr.* **6**, 159 (1977).
9. H. V. Kuhnlein, A. C. Chan, J. N. Thompson, and S. Nakai, Ooligan grease: A nutritious fat used by native people of coastal British Columbia. *J. Ethnobiol.* **2**, 154 (1982).
10. Meals for Millions Foundation, Southwest Program, *O'odham I:waki, wild greens of the desert people,* Meals for Millions Foundation, Tucson, 1980.
11. H. V. Kuhnlein, D. H. Calloway, and B. H. Harland, Composition of traditional Hopi foods. *J. Am. Diet. Assoc.* **75**, 37 (1979).
12. N. J. Turner, Indian Use of Shepherdia Canadensis, Soapberry, in Western North America. *Davidsonia* (U.B.C. Botanical Garden Publ.) **12**(1), 1 (1981).
13. R. A. Bye, Jr., Quelites—Ethnoecology of edible greens—Past, present and future. *J. Ethnobiol.* **1**, 109 (1981).

14. J. A. Duke, Nutritional values for crop diversification matrix. *Ecol. Food Nutr.* **6**, 39 (1977).

15. R. A. Bye, Jr. and I. Linares, The role of plants found in the Mexican markets and their importance in ethnobotanical studies. *J. Ethnobiol.* **3**, 1 (1983).

16. Panel of the Advisory Committee on Technology Innovation, National Research Council. *The Winged Bean. A High Protein Crop for the Tropics*, 2nd ed., National Academy Press, Washington, D.C., 1981.

17. J. R. K. Robson, R. I. Ford, K. V. Flannery, and J. E. Konlande, The nutritional significance of maize and teosinte. *Ecol. Food Nutr.* **4**, 243 (1976).

18. B. E. Nicholson, S. G. Harrison, G. B. Masefield, and M. Wallis, *The Oxford Book of Food Plants*, Oxford University Press, Oxford, U.K., 1971.

19. N. J. Turner, A gift for the taking: the untapped potential of some food plants of North American Native People. *Can. J. Bot.* **59**, 2331 (1981).

20. E. S. Sturtevant, *Sturtevant's Edible Plants of the World*, reprinted from the 1919 edition, edited by U. P. Hedrick, Dover, New York, 1972.

21. C. F. Saunders, *Edible and Useful Wild Plants of the United States and Canada*, Dover, New York, 1976.

22. E. E. Weatherbee and J. G. Bruce, *Edible Wild Plants of the Great Lakes Region*, University of Michigan, Ann Arbor, 1980.

23. A. F. Szczawinski and G. A. Hardy, *Guide to Common Edible Plants of British Columbia*, B.C. Provincial Museum Handbook No. 20, Victoria, 1971.

24. J. Burand, *Alaska's Game is Good Food*, Publ. 126, Cooperative Extension Service, University of Alaska, 1974.

25. P. Montagne, *The New Larousse Gastronomique*, Crown, New York, 1978.

26. E. A. Ellis and J. Simpkins, *Northern Cookbook*, Queens Printer, Ottawa, 1967.

27. I. S. Rombauer and M. R. Becker, *Joy of Cooking*, Allen and Son, Toronto, 1975.

28. Committee on Food Protection, National Research Council. *Toxicants Occurring Naturally in Foods*, National Academy of Sciences, Washington, D.C., 1973.

29. J. M. Kingsbury, *Poisonous Plants of the United States and Canada*, Prentice-Hall, Inc., Englewood Cliffs, N.J., 1964.

30. A. F. Szczawinski and N. J. Turner, *Edible Wild Greens of Canada*, National Museum of Natural Sciences, Ottawa, 1980.

31. N. J. Turner and A. F. Szczawinski, *Wild Coffee and Tea Substitutes of Canada*, National Museum of Natural Sciences, Ottawa, 1978.

32. N. J. Turner and A. F. Szczawinski, *Edible Wild Fruits and Nuts of Canada*, National Museum of Natural Sciences, Ottawa, 1979.

33. W. W. Leung, F. Burron, and C. Jardin, *Food Composition Table for Use in Africa*, FAO, Rome, 1968.

34. W. W. Leung, R. Butrum, F. H. Chang, M. N. Rao, and W. Polacchi, *Food Composition Table for Use in East Asia*, FAO, Rome, 1972.

35. W. Polacchi, J. S. McHargue, and B. P. Perloff, *Food Composition Tables for the Near East*, FAO, Rome, 1982.
36. W. W. Leung and M. Flores, *Food Composition Table for Use in Latin America*, INCAP-ICNND, 1961.
37. B. K. Watt and A. L. Merrill, *Composition of Foods*, Agriculture Handbook No. 8, Consumer and Food Economics Research Division, Agricultural Research Service, United States Department of Agriculture, Washington, D.C., 1963.
38. J. A. Pennington and H. N. Church, *Food Values of Portions Commonly Used*, 13th Ed., Harper and Row, Publishers, New York, 1980.
39. Health and Welfare Canada, *Nutrient Value of Some Common Foods*, Health Services and Promotion Branch and Health Protection Branch, Ottawa, 1979.
40. J. R. K. Robson and J. N. Elias, *The Nutritional Value of Indigenous Wild Plants: An Annotated Bibliography*, Whitston Publishing, Troy, N.Y., 1978.
41. E. Yanovsky and R. M. Kingsbury, Analysis of some Indian plant foods. *J. Assoc. Official Agric. Chem.* **21**, 648 (1938).
42. T. Arnason, R. J. Hebda, and T. Johns, Use of plants for food and medicine by native peoples of eastern Canada. *Can. J. Bot.* **59**, 2189 (1981).
43. D. H. Calloway, R. D. Giauque, and F. M. Costa, The superior mineral content of some American Indian foods in comparison to federally donated counterpart commodities. *Ecol. Food Nutr.* **3**, 203 (1974).
44. E. M. Benson, J. M. Peters, M. A. Edwards, and L. A. Logan, Nutritive values of wild edible plants of the Pacific Northwest. *J. Am. Diet. Assoc.* **62**, 143 (1973).
45. P. B. Keely, *Nutrient Composition of Selected Important Plant Foods of the Pre-contact Diet of the Northwest Native American Peoples*, M.S. Thesis, University of Washington, Department of Nutritional Sciences, 1980.
46. F. W. Martin and R. M. Ruberte, *Edible Leaves of the Tropics*, Published jointly by U.S. Agency for International Development and the Agriculture Research Service, Antillian College Press, Mayaguez, Puerto Rico, 1975.
47. W. W. Wainio and E. B. Forbes, The chemical composition of forest fruits and nuts from Pennsylvania. *J. Agr. Res.* **62**, 627 (1941).
48. G. P. Spinner and J. S. Bishop, Chemical analysis of some wildlife foods in Connecticut. *J. Wildlife Manage.* **14**, 175 (1950).
49. W. M. Beeson, H. R. Bird, E. W. Crompton, G. K. Davis, R. M. Forbes, L. E. Harris, L. E. Hanson, J. K. Loosli, J. E. Oldfeld, A. D. Tillman, J. R. Aitken, J. M. Bell, L. W. McElroy, W. J. Pigden, and W. D. Morrison, *Atlas of Nutritional Data on United States and Canadian Feeds*, National Academy of Sciences, Washington, D.C., 1971.
50. D. K. Brown, *Vitamin, Protein and Carbohydrate Content of Some Arctic Plants from the Fort Churchill, Manitoba Region*. Defense Research Northern Laboratory Tech. Paper No. 23, Defense Research Board, Dept. of National Defense, Ottawa, 1954.

51. T.M. Zennie and C.C. Ogzewalla, Ascorbic acid and vitamin A content of edible wild plants of Ohio and Kentucky, *Econ. Bot.* **31**, 76 (1977).
52. A. Johnston, L.M. Bezeau, and S. Amoliak, Chemical composition and in vitro digestibility of alpine tundra plants. *J. Wildlife Manage.* **32**, 773 (1968).
53. H.F. Drury and S.G. Smith, *Alaskan Wild Plants as an Emergency Food Source*, Fourth Alaskan Science Conf. Proceedings, 1953, p. 155.
54. T.R. King and H.E. McClure, Chemical composition of some American wild feedstuffs. *J. Agric. Res.* **69**, 33 (1944).
55. G.V. Mann, E.M. Scott, L.M. Hursch, C.A. Heller, J.B. Youmans, C.F. Consolazio, E.B. Bridgforth, A.A. Russel, and D.M. Silverman, The health and nutritional status of Alaskan Eskimos. *Am. J. Clin. Nutr.* **11**, 31 (1962).
56. M.G. MacPherson and E.G. Young, The chemical composition of marine algae. *Can. J. Res.* **27**, 73 (1949).
57. J.M. Navia, H. Lopez, M. Cimadevilla, E. Fernandez, A. Valiente, and I.D. Clement, Nutrient composition of Cuban foods, I. Foods of vegetable origin. *Food Res.* **20**, 97 (1955).
58. J.M. Navia, H. Lopez, M. Cimadevilla, E. Fernandez, A. Valiente, and I.D. Clement, Nutrient composition of Cuban foods, II. Foods of vegetable origin. *Food Res.* **22**, 131 (1957).
59. H. Lopez, J.M. Navia, D. Clement, and R.S. Harris, Nutrient composition of Cuban foods, III. Foods of vegetable origin. *J. Food Sci.* **28**, 600 (1963).
60. F.A. Farmer and H.R. Neilson, The caloric value of meats and fish of Northern Canada. *J. Can. Dietet. Assoc.* **28**, 174 (1967).
61. F.A. Farmer and H.R. Neilson, The nutritive value of canned meat and fish from Northern Canada. *J. Can. Diet. Assoc.* **31**, 102 (1970).
62. F.A. Farmer, M.L. Ho, and H.R. Neilson, Analysis of meats eaten by humans or fed to dogs in the Arctic. *J. Can. Diet. Assoc.* **32**, 137 (1971).
63. K. Hoppner, J.M. McLaughlan, B.G. Shah, J.N. Thompson, J. Beare-Rogers, J. Ellestad-Sayed, and O. Schaefer, Nutrient levels of some foods of Eskimos from Arctic Bay, N.W.T., Canada, *J. Am. Diet. Assoc.* **73**, 257 (1978).
64. J.D. Speth and K.A. Spielmann, Energy source, protein metabolism and hunter-gatherer subsistence strategies. *J. Anthrop. Archaeol.* **2**, 1 (1983).
65. J. Ramos Elorduy de Conconi, *Los Insectos como fuente de Proteinas en el Futuro*, Editorial Limusa, Mexico City, 1982.
66. Caribbean Food and Nutrition Institute, *Food Composition Tables for Use in the English-Speaking Caribbean*. P.O. Box 140, Kingston 7, Jamaica, 1974.
67. M. Murai, F. Pen, and C.D. Miller, *Some Tropical South Pacific Island Foods*, University of Hawaii Press, Honolulu, 1958.
68. E. Gibbons, *Stalking the Healthful Herbs*, David McKay Co., New York, 1966, p. 270.

69. H. V. Kuhnlein, N. J. Turner, and P. D. Kluckner, Nutritional significance of two important root foods (springbank clover and Pacific silverweed) used by native people of the coast of British Columbia. *Ecol. Food Nutr.* **12**, 89 (1982).

70. J. A. Pennington, *Dietary Nutrient Guide*, Avi Publishing, Westport, Conn., 1976.

71. R. Shosteck, How good are wild foods?, *The Mother Earth News* **60**, 111 (1979).

72. M. M. Tabekhia, R. B. Toma, and A. R. El-Mahdy, Effect of Egyptian cooking methods on total free oxalates and mineral contents of two leafy vegetables (Jew's mellow and purslane), *Nutr. Rep. Int.* **18**, 611 (1978).

73. J. Vengris, M. Drake, W. G. Colby, and J. Bart, Chemical composition of weeds and accompanying crop plants. *Agron. J.* **45**, 213 (1953).

74. G. C. Marten and R. N. Andersen, Forage nutritive value and palatability of 12 common annual weeds, *Crop Sci.* **15**, 821 (1975).

75. J. H. L. Truscott, W. Johnstone, T. Drake, J. VanHaarlem, and C. Thomson, *A Survey of the Ascorbic Acid Content of Fruits, Vegetables, and Some Native Plants Grown in Ontario, Canada*, Can. Counc. Nutr. Dept., National Health and Welfare, Ottawa, 1943.

76. H. V. Kuhnlein, The trace element content of indigenous salts compared with commercially refined substitutes. *Ecol. Food and Nutr.* **10**, 113 (1980).

ADDITIONAL RECENT REFERENCES

77. B. F. Ames, Dietary carcinogens and anticarcinogens. *Science* **221**, 1256 (1983).

78. People of K'san, *Gathering What the Great Nature Provided.* Douglas and McIntyre, Vancouver, B.C., 1981.

79. H. V. Kuhnlein, Traditional and contemporary Nuxalk Foods. *Nutr. Res.* (in press).

80. D. Lepofsky, N. J. Turner, and H. V. Kuhnlein. Determining the availability of traditional wild plant foods: an example of Nuxalk foods, Bella Coola, British Columbia. *Ecol. Food Nutr.* (in press).

81. H. H. Norton, E. S. Hunn, C. S. Martinsen, and P. B. Keely. Vegetable food products of the foraging economies of the Pacific Northwest. *Ecol. Food Nutr.* **14**, 219 (1984).

82. Nuxalk Food and Nutrition Program. *Nuxalk Food and Nutrition Handbook.* Malibu Printing, Richmond, B.C., 1984.

Cultural Nutrition

9

The Pursuit of Slenderness and Addiction to Self-Control

AN ANTHROPOLOGICAL INTERPRETATION OF EATING DISORDERS

MARGARET MACKENZIE, Ph.D., R.N.
Alcohol Research Group
School of Public Health
University of California, Berkeley

Address correspondence to Margaret Mackenzie, Ph.D., Alcohol Research Group, School of Public Health, University of California, Berkeley, California 94720.

ABSTRACT

What are eating disorders? How many individuals are affected? Who is vulnerable? Why mainly women? Why now? How are eating disorders related to obesity? How might they be treated? Can they be prevented? How could anthropology shed light on these questions? Fervor in the pursuit of slenderness is so persistent among the image-conscious members of contemporary affluent societies that health, beauty, media, and fashion seem insufficient to explain it. Adding to psychological and biological analyses the anthropological concepts of society, culture, and context—historical, economic, political, and familial—shows that fear of fatness, interpreted as caused by overeating and underexercising, is neither trivial nor unrealistic as one symbol of failure to achieve elemental moral virtues (for example, self-control, essential for self-confidence and access to high status). Research in California suggests anorexia and bulimia are points on a continuum from minor binges to addictive dieting, vomiting, and drug use. Prejudice against the obese appears unjustified because those overweight through genetics or metabolism may not, or may no longer, overeat. Obsession with eating usually is one manifestation of some other distress, for example, loss of love, which, after emergency nutritional care, needs attention but always in the context of remembering that the pathology lies partly in the cultural predispositions to excessive control and the social restrictions on upward mobility for those who are not slender.

WHAT ANTHROPOLOGICAL INTERPRETATION MIGHT ADD TO SCIENTIFIC EXPLANATION

Anthropology, with its concepts of culture, society, and context, can make some sense of aspects of human behavior that are puzzling and even unintelligible otherwise. It is probably necessary to invoke the context of social influence and cultural meaning to make any sense at all of why it is so overwhelmingly important to so many, especially women, to be thin. The zeal of the pursuit of slenderness is so remarkable that it hardly seems explicable solely on the grounds of promoting health, especially since the scientific evidence about the dangers of obesity is no longer so clear-cut as it once was. Health, with an emphasis on living longer and looking younger, certainly is a very powerful motive. Yet, even in concert with the influence of fashion and the media, it scarcely seems enough to account for a fear in contemporary affluent societies that is lived out as persistently, and talked about as incessantly, as is the fear of being fat, because of the intensity of the prejudice experienced by fat people in friendship, in employment, and even in medical care. It would seem that a sanction on fatness that is so extreme that some find themselves starving and vomiting compulsively in their attempt to avoid it must touch on something more elemental—some chord that the themes of health, fashion, and the media all restate, and in their recapitulation intensify, without themselves being the source of the prohibition.

One reason that the taboo on obesity may be so severe that it can precipitate compulsive eating, and does prompt discrimination against the fat, is that obesity is interpreted as a transgression against the basic cultural moral tenets of these societies. Obesity is seen as a failure in such cultural virtues as the responsibility to strive for self-control, willpower, rationality, competence, and productivity. Being fat is attributed to eating too much and/or exercising too little. Whatever the scientific evidence that genetics and metabolism, as well as the effects of chronic dieting and drug treatment, complicate this equation, there is a conviction that being fat means a loss of control of eating and a laziness in exercise. Those are cultural symbols suggesting moral shortcomings in self-discipline, perhaps the worst of all moral failures in social groups that bestow high status on those thought to have performed meritoriously through delayed gratification of impulses in pursuit of future goals.

In the context of abundant food supplies, where physical labor has become unnecessary, restraint in eating and effort in exercise may become symbols of social prestige. They can be interpreted as symbolic statements that luxurious foods and physical languor are such everyday affairs that there is no need to overindulge in festival foods or to lounge about as ordinary people do on special occasions. Eating only frugal portions of exquisite food in public becomes a metaphor for prosperity.

Restraint may be a symbol of those who count themselves civilized in many societies, but in those societies vulnerable to episodes of food scarcity, such as the South Pacific islands which may be laid waste overnight by a hurricane, that restraint is unlikely to be symbolized by refusing food, but rather in other metaphors, such as the mastery of the discipline of sacred rituals or the control of a political council. On the island of Tonga, for example, it is almost necessary for the king to be physically immense. His great size distinguishes him from commoners, who work all day growing food, part of which is given in tribute to the royal house. In fact, his stature and girth might be largely hereditary, but they are also cultural symbols of prosperity in a context where only a king can control enough food resources and labor supply to eat enough and do no physical labor so that he becomes fat.

In such a cultural context, where people of high social status are fat, it makes sense that it is difficult to convince someone that being fat is a sign of lack of refinement, or is unfashionable, dangerous to health, or even more implausibly, a symbol of moral failure. In the United States it is hard to convince someone otherwise. These are cultural and social matters, where medicine, media, and marketing are interpenetrated with meanings and metaphors whose source lies beyond their immediate boundaries. Nevertheless, to argue that it is necessary to interpret the fervor of the quest for control in the context of society and culture is not to argue that the science and the common sense are unnecessary or irrelevant; it is to claim that the levels of cultural and social context are a necessary, if not sufficient, part of any interpretation of human action and experience.

CULTURAL INTERPRETATION

The study of culture is the study of shared meanings and of the symbols in which they are expressed. Such meanings are shared in the social groups to which people belong, or wish to join, or even to reject. Although anthropologists work with individuals, their unit of analysis is not the individual idiosyncratic meaning, but rather the meanings that are more or less general in the society studied. Thus the anthropological perspective is only one facet of an interpretation, because a complete explanation would also need to include individual psychology and physiology to understand why some members of the society might be distressed about their eating patterns.

To say that cultural meanings are shared is not to claim that everyone accepts them or agrees with them. Instead, it is to say that most people are aware that they are issues in the society, whether or not they themselves have to deal with them; the fear of loss of control of eating may not worry them personally, but they are likely to be aware that it is an experience that many others have to struggle with daily.

SOCIAL ANALYSIS

The anthropological study of society is the study of patterns of social interaction and of social structure, from the fine-grained levels of the household to the wide canvas of the most encompassing influences and constraints on the group. The strengths of social anthropology that have something to offer in accounting for the vehement rejection of fatness in the executive and managerial occupations of affluent societies are its capacities to analyze social status, social mobility (both upward and downward), social control and social compliance, social conformity, stigma, prejudice, and social features of the access to scarce resources. Equally important are its studies of power and of the professions, and of who has the authority to define what will be included as knowledge in education. At the same time, anthropology has the theoretical framework to set these considerations in terms of the overall large-scale institutions of the society and of their dynamics. Any description of why so many people dread gaining weight if they want to be upwardly mobile in the United States would need to include, for example, the themes of the creation of the consumer, the marketing and advertising of food, and of slenderness, all at the same time, the dissemination of ideals of beauty through the selling of body image and of exercise, the use of anorectic models with figures similar to those of prepubertal males to display high fashion for women, the homogenization of society brought about by national media, and the sequences of scientific paradigms that characterize successive phases of research so that certain types of questions dominate during one period and are eclipsed during another—perhaps shaped by the cultural meanings that have filtered into the hypotheses unnoticed and unintended. If research on eating disorders should focus on such questions as the locus of control and restrained eating, it hardly seems possible that these issues would be entirely independent of the cultural moral issues specific to affluent societies that place a high value on striving for control, and that they might not validly be universally applicable.

CONTEXT

The anthropological focus on context is based on the axiom that what people think and do in any one sphere of their lives is inextricably connected with what they think and do in every other sphere, and with what has been embedded and distilled in history and tradition. This is sometimes called a holistic approach because it involves the study of social, cultural, and historical background to interpret whatever is the focus of the research. The concept of culture is not just one of isolated traits, usually irrational and peculiar, found scattered through any social group; rather, those traits will epitomize and encapsulate, repeat and reflect the warp of cultural meanings and the weft of the social dynamics that form the entire fabric of a society. These meanings and social features will vary slightly with differences in areas of experience and action. Nevertheless, they will be discernible as the various manifestations of a pervasive cultural or social tendency.

An elucidation of the historical context of attitudes to obesity in the United States includes the development in the nineteenth century of hybrid species in agriculture, of food processing and refrigeration, and of rail transport, so that abundant food became available to all. The paunch on the male and the commodious hips on the woman in middle age, which were taken as signs of respectability and prosperity, were no longer scarce. The symbols reversed: what became scarce metaphorically at the turn of the twentieth century was self-control instead of self-indulgence.

At the same time, the control of medicine passed from the hands of women healers into the realm of scientific medical schools in the universities. The focus shifted towards experimentation and measurement; away from acute to what was defined as chronic disease. Responsibility for health proceeded from public hygiene to private responsibility for compliance with professional recommendations regarding drug treatment and personal behavior of the individual.

Another consideration is the history of the definition of problems now defined as medical. Originally, gluttony was the sin of eating too much. To be a sin it had to entail a deliberate decision; any impairment of free choice would have mitigated the evil. Today, what is perceived as excessive eating has become defined as an illness, at least partly from the compassionate intention of removing the moral stigma attached to it, and partly because medicine has taken over from institutionalized religion, at least to some extent, in the province of morals in a secular modern world.

The price paid for the medicalization of moral problems, however, is high. The cost in exchange for removing the stigma of sin is accepting the diagnosis of inadequate willpower; instead of having a choice to eat, the patients are now defined as having a loss of control over their eating. There are few wounds to rival that of being seen as incompetent in achieving moral restraint. This is a psychodeterminism of deviance.

The experience of loss of control of eating may be indeed real to a person; it may in fact occur. What is not clear is the extent to which such loss of control is a consequence of a cultural context that has almost no limit on the amount of control over eating expected from any individual.

In another shift motivated by a humane intent to lessen the stigma attached to shortcomings of self-discipline attributed to a person with disrupted eating patterns in this psychosomatic model, another theory regarding the cause is appearing; it might be called the "neosomatic" because it is a theory that returns the cause to the body and the brain, away from the mind and the will. It locates the disturbance in the physiological constitution of a person, focusing on such features as abnormalities in enzymes, hormones, or the release of neurotransmitters, the chemical messengers in the brain. Such aberrations are not regarded as accessible to conscious control. Thus, people may be impelled to overeat, not because they have weak wills, but, for example, because the level at which their appetite control mechanisms are set causes them to crave carbohydrates. Eating carbohydrates stimulates the production of insulin; insulin allows the level of tryptophan to rise; tryptophan enhances the release of the neurotransmitter serotonin in the brain, which in turn leads to the suppression of carbohydrate intake. The hypothesis is that those who crave carbohydrate have an abnormally high threshold for serotonin levels. It is hardly surprising that a proposed treatment would be the use of drugs that enhance serotonin release, which are believed to suppress appetite by decreasing the desire for carbohydrate (1).

Such theories are humane because they blame the victim less than theories that attribute inappropriate eating habits to conscious decision. The price paid for accepting a neosomatic abnormality, such as a neurochemical malfunction, is that one concedes to a definition of disability that is possibly permanent. Nevertheless, such theories recognize individual difference. They can also accommodate putative differences between eating disorders and obesity, without always attributing fatness to overeating and underexercise. Obesity can be discussed in terms of the increased efficiency of the body by the decreased consumption of oxygen, for instance, or in terms of lower thermogenesis—the decreased production of heat in the metabolism of food. Nevertheless, although it appears that the adverse moral judgments would be dissolved by attributing eating binges and fatness to physical causes, some connotations of moral weakness remain, especially when overtones of pleasure might be involved. There is some implication that the serotonin levels sought by the carbohydrate cravers might be related to the activation of endorphins, the body's natural opiates that relieve pain. And, too often, unintentionally, the Protestant Ethic seems to be projected onto animals: rats given palatable chow always appear to eat more than rats fed the regular laboratory diet. One is left with an impression that the palatable is problematic.

To trace the cycles of the different frameworks in which research on eating or obesity has been conceived from the somatic to the psychosomatic and back to the neosomatic is not to claim that such research is invalid; it is only to say that the organizing metaphors we choose or use for conceptualizing the questions are not entirely independent of cultural meaning and historical influence. Because we are people, and we do not stop being human when we do research, it is inevitable that the hypotheses may contain traces of social, cultural, and historical imprints. Such trails may be ineradicable, but they can be at least partially recognized if never entirely eliminated.

The methods of anthropological research are even more open to the influence of the anthropologist's own background than are those of science. Because we are humans studying a human world, our own aspiration to abstract objectivity is the pursuit of an illusion. The people we study manage us by the access they permit us to their lives. They assign us roles in their society. We negotiate as well as we can for the status we wish to assume. In such a context, we may become permanent blots on the landscape, but never flies on the wall; the people rarely forget we are there and seldom behave as if we are not. Just because we are doing field work, we cannot suddenly shed our own history and culture—everything we are as people—although we can seek to identify our social heritage and our personal character and take account of them. Everything we see and hear is filtered through our social lenses and translated into our cultural categories. Because the result is an interpretation, such an argument is not a proof; it is of course open to alternative interpretations. In the end, the criterion for choosing which interpretation is more fruitful comes down to which one makes more sense of the unintelligible symbols and the puzzling actions, for the sizes of the samples anthropologists interview seldom are large enough to satisfy the statistician. The elucidation of deeply held convictions and of subtle distinctions takes months and even years of close contact, usually with small numbers of people. This is particularly true since the anthropologist is often fumbling in a foreign language and the research may raise painful questions to which serious answers would be given only in a context of mutual trust and respect that take a long time to build.

In such circumstances it is understandable that anthropological interpretations might be discredited as impressionistic generalizations. Nevertheless, if reliability is defined as being able to get another observer to replicate about 50% of the results, it would seem possible that another anthropologist able to fit into the same social niche as the first in the society studied, and equipped with similar theoretical training, might get such overlap in results. One clue that the interpretation may be authentic is to submit it to the people studied and ask for their reaction. If they recognize it as making sense of their own lives, even in a way they may not have articulated for themselves before, then the interpretation probably is tenable.

The interpretations made here are based on 10 years of research in California studying eating and weight; 93 people have been interviewed, some many times, formally and informally, and studied by participant observation in clinical settings for weight reduction, anorexia nervosa, bulimia, and distressed eating. Approximately 1000 more have sought me out to talk about their theories or their problems related to eating and/or weight because they knew I was studying them. None of this was in formal treatment programs. Beyond that, nutritionists, psychologists, counselors, and fat activists have discussed their thinking with me. The comparative perspective that highlights attitudes and actions in the United States comes from field work on nutrition and health in three South Pacific islands: Savai'i in Western Samoa, Malekula in Vanuatu, and Rarotonga in the Cook Islands.

What such research can contribute is a perspective on the social and cultural context of the scientific investigations and the treatment programs, because inevitably the social and cultural currents of the time infiltrate even the most controlled laboratory. Hypotheses may be tested immaculately once they are formulated, and clinical trials may be conducted scrupulously, but it is in the choice of research questions, in the formulation of the hypotheses themselves, that the social currents and the cultural concerns penetrate.

WHAT ARE EATING DISORDERS?

The definitions of diagnostic criteria for eating disorders are specified in the Diagnostic and Statistical Manual of Mental Disorders, Third Edition, published in 1980, widely referred to as DSM-III (2). It lays out a set of criteria for anorexia nervosa and bulimia, assigning features that do not conform to either but appear related, to the category of borderline personality disorders. Anorexia nervosa, category 307.10, is classified as an intense fear of becoming obese which does not diminish as weight loss progresses; as a disturbance of body image, for example, feeling fat even when emaciated; as a weight loss of at least 25% of original body weight; as a refusal to maintain body weight over a minimal normal weight for age and height; and as a weight loss that cannot be accounted for by a known physical illness. Bulimia, category

307.51, is defined as recurrent episodes of binge eating, that is, rapid consumption of a large amount of food in a discrete period of time, usually less than two hours. At least three of the following criteria must occur to meet the classification: (1) consumption of high-caloric, easily ingested food during a binge; (2) inconspicuous eating during a binge; (3) termination of such eating episodes by abdominal pain, sleep, social interruption, or self-induced vomiting; (4) repeated attempts to lose weight by severely restricted diets, self-induced vomiting, or use of cathartics and/or diuretics; and (5) frequent weight fluctuations greater than 10 pounds due to alternating binges and fasts. In addition, there must be awareness that the eating pattern is abnormal, fear of not being able to stop eating voluntarily, depressed mood and self-deprecating thoughts following eating binges, and the bulimic episodes must not be due to anorexia nervosa or any known physical disorder.

With the publication of DSM-III, diagnosis epitomizes part of the move to a neosomatic phase from the psychosomatic one that had characterized much of medical science and psychiatry. The symptoms are usually discrete elements. The diagnostic criteria are usually separable categories, thus necessitating further categories to which the ambiguous symptoms can be consigned. The criteria usually are externally observable symptoms. All of the diagnoses are capable of being coded.

Such a situation seems not only perfectly reasonable, but important and necessary in an age of computing and the compilation of internationally comparable statistics. Nevertheless, these features do reflect the priorities of our time, and they neglect what might have been the priorities of another time. There is no room for a continuum of symptoms in a system of discrete categories that can be specified precisely, where the remainder that do not conform are assigned to a residual category. Yet the essence of eating disorders may be that they are a continuum, and that having to categorize them into discrete conditions may conceal their origin, process, and even some clues for their solution.

The anthropological interviews in California with people who come from all over the United States, from Canada, and from Western Europe and its former colonies, suggest that concern about eating may be a nearly predictable response to the social pressures and cultural meanings among contemporary elites, especially for women. The material revealed that, in a sense, only the lucky ones escape—lucky by the birth of a metabolism and a constitution that makes neither the issue of eating nor the fact of fat a problem. Such people are a minority who may be psychologically sturdy because they are physically fortunate by the present ideals for body size. For the rest, fearful of becoming fat either because of genetic heritage or fearful of losing control of eating (which precipitates the very fact it dreads—to go on a diet is to cause compulsive eating) there is a risk of a continuum of minor or massive losses of control of eating occasionally or often. What is feared may range from an extra glass of orange juice to thousands of calories from foods usually forbidden as dangerously pleasurable and nutritionally tabooed. The exhortations of nutrition education may get deflected and distorted in desperate efforts to impose a control that is unrealistically austere, where pleasure is nearly always problematic.

What is at issue much of the time, it seems to me, is a response to a cultural context in which self-control is the pinnacle of the acceptance of oneself and of others as worthwhile people. Again and again, the solution pursued—complete control of impulses to eat foods defined as pleasurable but nutritionally valueless—itself becomes the problem. Until the taboo on these foods is removed, they retain eternally their risk of ruin. Once one bite is taken, the eating may never stop. The model of addiction has been adopted from concepts of the loss of control of drugs such as heroin and alcohol. The problem is that abstinence from eating is not possible, although about half of anorectics attempt it. For the rest, for the bulimics, and for many more people in minor ways, the very attempt to gain complete control seems connected to the creation of a virtual obsession with what is banned.

To define such behavior into separate categories based on mainly physical criteria, such as weight loss, makes sense. A starving anorectic may urgently need heroic measures to forestall imminent death. Such categories conceal the continuum of the concerns about loss of control that characterize people's own accounts of their problems. They favor calories that can be counted but which are not the real core of the problem—a binge of half a sandwich may distress one person nearly as much as one of five thousand calories distresses another. Agony may be completely independent of amounts eaten. People who do not conform to the diagnostic criteria may remain neglected in their distress because their binges are too mild to be defined as meriting treatment. Ironically, they may be the ones most able to be helped. At the same time, the literature is deflected towards the most extreme cases, not only because the conditions may be life-threatening but because the others do not qualify for diagnosis and description.

The implications of the diagnostic categories go further. By defining certain behaviors as deviant and individual, thus as falling into the province of medical treatment, we may make private problems of what are in fact public issues. The pathology may lie in the cultural meanings to which the starving, the compulsive dieting, the vomiting, and certainly the concern about loss of control could be claimed to be a realistic response, especially given the very real consequences of being fat and prejudiced against in employment, in promotion, in marriage, in admission to medical school, and even in adopting children.

Of course it is urgent to help people distressed about their loss of control, and even in danger of dying from their dieting, by giving them medical treatment. Of course it is reasonable to want to give them a sense of control in their lives, a sense of taking charge of themselves, a sense of being able to survive independently as autonomous beings able to resist the pressures of parents and society. But concealed in this compassionate psychological assertiveness training are cultural values about control and autonomy which may themselves be unrealistic and more in need of change than the people who seek treatment. Behavioral methods used in conjunction with nutritional programs may also show that part of the treatment is attempting to inculcate more control when the problem may already be one of sabotage by attempts at overcontrol.

The cultural symbols and the social facts may be part of the cause, and attention to them might dissolve some of the symptoms. Although we seldom address issues of social and cultural change because the task seems utterly overwhelming, that does not mean that we should forget other sources of pathology than the individual or, conversely, retreat to reducing the issues entirely to biological determinism when the individual psychological model wavers. Although we do not have the knowledge or capacity to change the culture singlehandedly, we can continue to analyze it critically and work to change it together. There are implications of this position that can help the individual meanwhile.

Paradoxically, it may be only when a person stops dieting and dares to permit pleasure that the specter of loss of control in eating evaporates! Such a prescription is not easy to follow when 10, 20, or even 40 years may have been spent doing the opposite, but there are people who have found that it stopped their compulsive eating. Nevertheless, for many the terror that they may have to endure episodes of eating binges, and even weight gain, sabotages their courage to relinquish their preoccupation with control. For some, membership in a group such as Overeaters Anonymous does stop their compulsive eating, but for others whose goal is to lose weight, such a program based on the treatment of addictive eating may be self-defeating if they do not already suffer from eating binges. Some have found they start compulsive eating in circumstances where it is made problematic.

Equally difficult, and less immediately realistic for those most distressed about their eating, is the injunction to accept a larger body size when moral worth and acceptable achievement are symbolized by slenderness.

Beyond solace for the present pain, what may be needed most is a critique of the passion to comply with a culture that values striving for a good perceived as external to a person, always to be attained in the future by eliminating patterns in the present. Instead of defining good as already present within a person, of believing that people are worthy of self-respect and respect from others independently of the amount of fat on their bodies, people aspiring to contemporary elites encounter the heritage of beliefs in Original Sin, the exile from Paradise, the distrust of bodily impulses that culminated in a dualism with a mind separate from and superior to the body, and then a mind divided into higher reason and potentially chaotic emotions that must be mastered by intellect.

Such an ideology of control paradoxically symbolizes freedom! The meaning of liberty is the capacity of freedom to choose, and people are not free if they are unable to choose to stop eating. The subjugation of impulses to indulge oneself by eating is therefore not a trivial matter to be dismissed as a symptom of the trite and vain concerns of women with nothing better to think about.

What is at stake is human nature and the fundamental moral ideals of the culture. What is also at stake is social access to scarce resources in which it seems the prize goes to the perfect, when one of the few areas accessible to individual control is the amount of fat on the body. If one could just get enough control of eating and exercise, then there is a chance of being selected from all the other candidates for the job, or the friendship. It is a magical quest.

These are hardly only nutritional issues. Nutrition is merely the surface, even the mask, of deeper distress about individual character that may have a cultural and social origin. Nutrition may not be involved at all if the issue is one of weight without eating disorders, unless a person inclined by metabolism to a larger size than the ideal is trapped into eating problems by the sanctions of others and the internalization of oppression in deviating from the ideals.

To answer the question of what eating disorders are has involved a journey into social and cultural context. Yet, an anthropological answer neglects the meanings that disrupted eating does have in individual psychopathology. Certainly the college students interviewed who were caught in cycles of binge eating and vomiting several times a day, in the use of diuretics and diet pills, in the compulsive use of laxatives and sometimes amphetamines, did have histories of attempted suicide, of depression, of social isolation. Yet, every one who had such severe symptoms also came from family situations with deeply disturbed communication patterns, often with double-binds; where fat phobia was intense in the parents, especially their fathers; and where repression of emotions was inculcated so that a limited repertoire of feelings was instilled. The students felt that they were not entitled to be angry or depressed or sad because they were warm, dry, and well-fed. They came from comfortable financial backgrounds, they went to good schools, they had their own bedrooms. What right had they to feel depressed?

Even this individual psychopathology seemed to have been partly rooted in family psychodynamics. Surprising were the relations with their fathers reported by anorectic daughters: a perception of an affectionate relationship suddenly withdrawn when the girl reached puberty. "I thought that if I grew small enough he would love me again!" wept one anorectic during an interview. Instead of one common interpretation of anorectics as individuals who begin at puberty to starve to avoid sexual relationships with men, these interviews revealed a desire to stay a child to remain close to a father. In these situations the mothers were often bystanders unable to bring themselves to intervene and equip their daughters to handle the interaction differently, perhaps because they could not cope with it themselves. Sometimes there was a history of incest.

Because those students interviewed who had the most severe symptoms also had deeply disrupted family dynamics, again the questions are raised of how much the individual is to be defined as deviant, and how much the illness lies in the social dynamics, when the adolescent is the one who manifests the symptoms defined as pathological, while the communication patterns are not visible to outsiders. Such an interpretation is so similar to the theories of adolescent schizophrenia formulated first by Bateson (3) that it must be emphasized that there was no hypothesis at all about such a pattern before the research began. It emerged from the results.

All of these students, and all of the people with eating disorders, had very high expectations of themselves. Their families placed extremely high goals before them. Such aspirations had often been achieved academically; the students interviewed were "A" students in a highly ranked university. Yet, they were never satisfied with their own performance, and their control of eating and weight came to symbolize the performance that would ultimately be accepted as the only truly worthwhile one. Until they felt in complete control of their eating and their weight, they believed that they did not really deserve credit for their achievements.

This is a context of excessive conformity. The problem is not compliance, but overcompliance with cultural ideals. For this reason, people who have independent minds, who refuse to conform, or who are eccentric, are less vulnerable. By no means is it clear-cut to call an individual ill because of their over conformity to a culture. This is tantamount to blaming a child for being too good, and to put the responsibility on that child for being able to judge precisely the point beyond which obedience becomes deviance.

It would seem clear that not everyone is vulnerable to finding herself or himself in this plight, because not all family psychodynamics are so disrupted, nor all aspirations so high, nor all feelings so disapproved. Yet, those who are vulnerable are not only the already affluent. Although most of the people interviewed were women, mostly white, mostly with some college education, and mostly financially comfortable, there were men as severely distressed as women, there were ethnic minorities, some were poor, and some had no higher education.

The core of the issue seems to be aspiration to high achievement and high status employment in societies where such high rank (defined by socioeconomic status) is perceived as scarce. This is held in a context of distrust of bodily impulses and a reverence for reason at the expense of emotion, with a concept of external good to be attained in a future through elimination of habits disapproved in the present.

The quest is one of ascetic achievement paradoxically occurring in a context of consumerism. It is one of ambivalence, ambiguity, and conflict about pleasure where pleasure seems ever-available but unreliably controllable. Women may be more vulnerable because traditionally the ascetic achievements accessible to them have been mostly related to controlling their size and preserving their youthful appearance. In a megasociety where people no longer can know one another face to face, personal criteria of evaluation, such as being aware that in private life someone is a superb mother, disappear. They are replaced by publicly visible impersonal criteria—such as fat on the hips. Only too often does it seem legitimate to assume that a fat woman has problems: if she cannot get her life together enough to get slim, then she probably could not organize her work well enough to be worth employing. Such thinking does not take account of the moral meaning attributed to a physical feature, a meaning that may have no rational or logical connection at all.

Men have had access to the workplace where they can demonstrate high performance through profits, sales, or books published. In a sense, women sometimes have become a commodity in this sphere; if a man brings a fat wife to the executive cocktail party, he is assumed to be a loser. Any competent man, the thinking goes, would have been able to obtain a wife who could keep slim.

Women are moving into the managerial workplace only recently, but the emphasis on their image has remained. Now there is a rejection of the "earth mother" in favor of the symbols of competence and performance—streamlined lean efficiency with the fat cut out. The symbols of control have intensified instead of weakened. As the world economy has floundered, and the traditional elites find their customary stability threatened, the perception of scarcity has aggravated the competition to enter and remain in managerial and executive status. In doing so, women have adopted many male symbols instead of establishing new ones of their own. For as Weber saw in *The Protestant Ethic and the Spirit of Capitalism* (4), the symbols underlying the Protestant Ethic are the same symbols that underlie free enterprise: the basis of capitalism is the ability to make contracts with reliable, competent, efficient individuals who are self-disciplined and morally responsible in a rational marketplace with a disciplined workforce. Thus, the cultural meanings that are at stake in being slim are the same cultural meanings that are at stake in the workplace. The pursuit of slenderness is not only about human nature, it is also about the relationship of the individual to work in society. No wonder the concern about controlling size through controlling eating is so passionate!

WHAT NUMBERS ARE INVOLVED?

An argument has been made here that eating disorders are better considered a continuum from minor to catastrophic losses of control of eating, ranging through to compulsive use of vomiting, laxatives, and other drugs. The data from surveys do not address the numbers affected by these problems. The surveys have focused on the discrete conditions of bulimia and anorexia nervosa, although sometimes they have included dieting. Within those categories, the definitions have varied, especially of bulimia, which can sometimes coincide with DSM-III, but sometimes is defined more stringently, such as by the number of calories consumed, or by the definite presence of vomiting. The latter may sometimes also be called bulimarexia.

Taking account of these variations, nevertheless there is a stunning congruence in the percentages of college students defined as bulimic. Again and again, about 11–14% of students have been defined as bulimic, 5% of them male. Of those defined as bulimic, 10% have been classified as vomiting compulsively and chronically. There is a reported association between vomiting and the use of drugs. If people vomit, they are more likely to be using diet pills, amphetamines, laxatives, diuretics, and other drugs, such as alcohol. For example, in a study at the University of California, Berkeley, surveying 689 undergraduates in their classes, Nevo found that 14% of the Caucasian women fitted her definition of bulimia; 40% of the Caucasian women binged on food at least once a month, 50% tried to lose weight at least once a month, and 60% worried a great deal about their weight. Of those with bulimia, 11% purged by vomiting. Dieting and weight concerns were highly correlated and close to being normally distributed (5). In another study on a college campus, Halmi et al. defined 13% of a sample of 355 as bulimic; 87% of the bulimics were women, 13% men. Of the bulimics, 10% were vomiting (6).

Do these data indicate a problem that should be taken seriously? My own answer is yes, because of the distress that so many young people are suffering, especially because there is so much binge eating reported, and binges indicate concern and sometimes even terror. Problems that are reported as nearly normally distributed show widespread pain, and even raise the question again of where the pathology lies. If everyone has an illness, is it then an illness or is it normal? Anthropologists in the Pacific are familiar with societies that did not see yaws, for example, as an illness because it was so common. Deeper than the question of what counts as an abnormality and what as normality is the issue that such common symptoms suggest: could the genesis lie partly in pathology that is inherent potentially in cultural and social themes? Facts of social status and symbols of cultural ideals may be part of the problem. Symbols may be as infectious as the microorganisms that cause yaws!

The survey data indicate that worries about eating are not restricted to people of college age. In a mail questionnaire distributed to respondents in 35 states in the United States, the National Association of Anorexia Nervosa and Associated Disorders found that of 1400 respondents self-diagnosed as anorectic or bulimic, 1.8% were aged over 50, 2.7% were 40–49, and 20.5% were 30–39: that is, 25% were over 30 (7). Such data suggest, reinforcing the data from anthropological interviews, that this is not a new problem. Women in their forties report occasionally that they have been binging and vomiting daily for 15 to 20 years. College students in the anthropological interviews reported that they began dieting in junior high school. By the beginning of high school, they had begun compulsive dieting. Some of them began vomiting soon afterwards; others did not vomit until they reached college. What may be new is the willingness to seek help for their problems, and thus the attention paid to them in the research and treatment literature. But there is no way of telling how much such attention has caused the conditions to increase, especially in the media, where people have become concerned about their own contribution to the problems.

Anorexia nervosa has attracted attention longer than bulimia. One rule of thumb has been that about 20% of college students suffer from it, and about 20% of those are likely to die. Half of the anorectics are likely to lose weight by starvation; the other half by alternate binging and vomiting, interrupted by cycles of starvation. In another college campus study done by Cusin and Svendsen and reported in the magazine *Ms*, in a sample of 944 sorority women, 38 upper-level dance majors, and 244 regular college coeds, 9% of the coeds, 16% of the sorority women, and 23% of the dance majors suffered from symptoms of anorexia nervosa (8). Again, social issues are raised: commonly dancers, actresses, athletes, and gymnasts simply cannot find employment unless their weight approaches the level of emaciation. It is at least partly understandable that they succumb to anorexia nervosa when their lifelong dreams are at stake.

While anorectics are easily detectable because of their visible emaciation, some of their other symptoms may not be visible. They tend to suffer extremely from feeling cold because of starvation. Their bodies become covered often with fine downy hair. They display an obsession with food by cooking gourmet meals for their households while they dine on raw cauliflower themselves. Very commonly they will exercise instead of appearing at lunch or dinner, announcing that they have had their meals elsewhere. Bulimics, on the other hand, may eat normally, or with great restraint, at meals they have with other people—except at pot-luck dinners, where the binging may be public. They too may suffer from the cold, wearing hats and gloves on a sunny warm day. Usually they do not appear at all emaciated if they are not anorectic by weight, and they may appear cheerful and competent. Sometimes, however, their skins may be affected with acne and their eyes reddened from blood vessels burst from vomiting. Their knuckles may show abrasions from vomiting inducing by putting their hands down their throats, and their teeth may be losing enamel from being bathed in the hydrochloric acid regurgitated from their stomachs along with the food. Their salivary glands may be swollen, as in mumps. They are vulnerable to rupture of the esophagus, not to mention sore throats from vomiting. They may run a risk of rupture of the stomach. If they are using laxatives, they may suffer from rectal bleeding. For all the appearance of being in charge of their lives on the surface, underneath they may be terrified. Nevertheless, they may be reluctant to seek treatment; nothing could be more appalling than to have the vomiting cured and to be left with the binging and the risk of the obesity about which they have a phobia.

But, such symptomatology applies again to the discrete and extreme cases classified as bulimia and anorexia. It diverts attention from those whose symptoms do not become physically discernible, but whose behavior may be anorectic or bulimic in the sense of compulsive eating and dieting that does not reach the level of emaciation. The distress lies in the behavior, and such behavior may indeed occur at any weight. It may also be inculcated by some dietary treatments, which in their severity mimic the very symptoms here defined as the problems.

DISCUSSION: WHAT CAN BE DONE?

Consistent with the anthropological focus of the paper, any statement about what practical implications this analysis might have begins with the reminder that this is an anthropological view and not a psychological, medical, or nutritional one. The province of anthropology, therefore, means that any discussion of what might be done to prevent or to treat a person worried about weight and obsessed with controlling eating might make a plea to remember that the culture of social elites in contemporary affluent societies is based on a context of striving for control and rewarding achievements reckoned to have required self-discipline. People who do not fulfill these criteria are treated with prejudice and do not have easy access to social privilege. In such a context, it is understandable that when fatness acquires a meaning of failure to achieve these virtues, people might become preoccupied with slenderness. If they associate obesity with eating and the neglect of exercise, they may get trapped in compulsive attempts to diet, and even in vomiting, as well as in obsessive exercise, particularly if they are women who see their access to prestigious positions as problematic. In such circumstances, one form of treatment is to treat the society and the culture by social and cultural change. Such change forms the background that needs to be remembered in treating any individual. If change seems impossible when one is faced with an individual caught deeply in the problems, the consciousness of the social and cultural influences is a reminder that the distressed person does not need to be defined as a freak, but rather as someone extremely responsive to social pressures. And in these societies women have been so trained.

A critical attitude to the social and cultural correlations of eating disorders nevertheless must not obscure the diversity of the problems of the people who suffer from the conditions. While the context of control forms the very backdrop for people's experience and aspirations, everyone has an individual history, a different family, and particular goals. What is manifest as disrupted eating is only the entry point to the problems that a person is trying to handle in living. If the entry is nutritional, and the context is social and cultural, then the focus of treatment still needs centrally to be psychological—once the crisis is no longer life-threatening, as in the emergency refeeding of a severe anorectic. It is nearly universal that the surface problem is merely the mask for others that would be even more agonizing to face than the one that is manifest, no matter how distressing that seems to be. Coping with the starving and purging will be likely to reveal someone who is ill at ease with anger, frustration, doubt, and sadness; one who is suffering from separation from parents and loss of love, whose concept of self is fragmented into elements that must be improved and others that must be eradicated.

Whatever the problems, they will be diverse, and individual attention to the specific person is essential. While drugs such as antidepressants, anticonvulsants, and the monoamine oxidase inhibitors may in fact stop the binge-eating, it is not clear that they solve the underlying problems. Apart from the side effects of drugs, the person who is an "A" student is not likely to be enthusiastic about sacrificing mental acuity for the tranquilizing effect of medication.

For some, the paradoxical treatment of persuading them to eat the foods formerly forbidden may work. Instead of a healthy diet, what they may need in the short run, so that they can eventually eat foods that are good for them, is to be persuaded to eat foods that are defined as bad! That is, until such foods as chocolate, candies, and ice cream have the power taken away from them by being made permissible, it may be impossible for someone to stop eating them.

Such strategies alone will rarely be enough, even for a person whose binges are occasional and minor. For them, it may be necessary to debunk the goal of eternal control, but it may also be essential to identify when the binges occur, and to find responses that distress them less. Many binges occur as a result of frustration with an employer or a lover. It may not be possible to express one's disapproval to an employer in a scarce job-market, or to risk losing a lover, but there may be less disturbing ways to handle the frustration than by eating.

Most of the people who suffer from eating disorders are dissatisfied with their bodies. They have a poor body image and they have low self-esteem. Some of the most effective help may come from teaching them to have more self-respect for their minds and their bodies.

The ideal goal would seem to be to have people living in the society who are able to survive its pressures as they work to change them, and to exorcize the extreme slenderness that at present saps so many people's energy and sanity. If people could be relieved of the self-condemnation and its consequences, think what they could achieve and how they could live!

What, then, might be done to prevent the damage that has been done already from being passed on to our children? The first of all principles is to love them—to love them simply for who they are as they are, independently of what they have achieved or how much they weigh. No one ever succeeds by attack, and children made to feel tortured by criticism of dissatisfied adults may have eating problems created where none existed earlier. Beyond that, making an issue of weight—threatening that they may not go back to school if they do not gain weight, or if they do not lose it—does not help. The very obsession that one seeks to remove may be intensified by such action. If people show signs of having an eating problem, then the best strategy is to find out what else might be wrong in their lives. Could they be frightened of losing love? Are they being threatened with incest? Or are they simply being told they are too fat? It is important to remember that adult weight cannot reliably be predicted until the age of four, and that if a child is fat at that age, he is likely to remain fat. In such circumstances, the best that one might do for those children is to equip them to live in a society where they will be subjected to prejudice (9). Making an issue of foods defined as pleasurable, and usually given as rewards but withheld from fat children, sets fat children into the groove of coming into impossible conflict with pleasure and eating; it almost creates an eating disorder. Such actions can occur with children of average size as well if a lower ideal weight is held out to them as a goal. Associating exercise with pleasure early in childhood is a true gift to a child. If activity is a treat and not a chore, then the child is likely to continue exercise into adulthood.

In the anthropological interviews, the students said again and again that they did not feel entitled to be depressed. It was as if in being told that they were fortunate to have a financially comfortable childhood, they were also being told that they must always present a face of cheerfulness, competence, and control. In such circumstances, they were scarcely able to discriminate feelings of anger, confusion, doubt, frustration; they had a limited repertoire of emotions. Instead of encouraging children always to be cheerful, we may be doing them a kindness to allow them to experience sadness when they are sad, doubt when they are confused, and rage when they are angry, no matter how uncomfortable it is for those around them. Unless they are able to experience their emotions, they may respond to every threatening feeling by eating, or drinking alcohol, or using drugs, or some other form of compulsive behavior. But, beyond all the specific instructions, the first strategy for prevention is to love and support them for who they are as they are now.

ACKNOWLEDGMENTS

The funds on which this research was based were Biomedical Sciences Grants from the University of California, Berkeley, in 1974; Committee on Research Funds from the University of California, Berkeley, 1974–1981; Center for Field Research for research in Western Samoa 1976; Public Health Service, Department of Health, Education and Welfare 1981–1983; and Damien Family Foundation 1983. The author wishes to thank the participants in the studies of obesity and of eating disorders in California and in Western Samoa, and the people not being studied formally who volunteered ideas and information.

REFERENCES

1. R. J. Wurtman, Behavioral effects of nutrients. *Lancet* **1**, 1145–47 (1983).
2. *Diagnostic and Statistical Manual of Mental Disorders*, 3rd. ed. American Psychiatric Association, Washington, D.C., 1980.
3. G. Bateson, D. D. Jackson, J. Haley, and J. H. Weakland, Toward a theory of schizophrenia. *Behav. Sci.* **I** (4), 1956. Reprinted in G. Bateson, *Steps to an Ecology of Mind*, Ballantine, New York, 1972, pp. 201–227.
4. M. Weber, *The Protestant Ethic and the Spirit of Capitalism* (1904). English translation by Talcott Parsons. Charles Scribner's Sons, New York, 1958.
5. S. Nevo, *Eating Patterns and Personality Characteristics of Bulimic and Overweight Women.* Ph.D. dissertation, University of California, Berkeley, Department of Psychology, 1982.
6. K. A. Halmi et al. Binge-eating and vomiting: A survey of a college population. *Psychological Medicine* **11** (4), 697–706 (1981).
7. National Association of Anorexia Nervosa and Associated Disorders, *Survey.* Highland Park, Ill., 1981.
8. J. Cusin and D. Svendsen. In S. Squire, Is the binge–purge cycle catching? *Ms*, pp. 41–46, October 1983.
9. P. Crawford, Obesity prognosis: A longitudinal study of children aged six months to nine years. Pending publication.

10
Social and Cultural Determinants of Breastfeeding in the United States

SARAH E. SAMUELS, Dr.P.H.
PEW Fellow/Nutritionist
Institute for Health Policy Studies
School of Medicine
University of California, San Francisco

Address correspondence to Sarah E. Samuels, Dr.P.H., PEW Fellow, Institute for Health Policy Studies, School of Medicine, 1326 Third Ave., University of California, San Francisco, California 94143.

ABSTRACT

Current research on trends and social and cultural obstacles to breastfeeding are reviewed in this chapter. In recent years there has been a noticeable increase in the incidence of breastfeeding in the United States. But, despite this increase, many women stop breastfeeding during the early postpartum weeks. Research has shown that white, middle-class, well-educated women are most likely to choose to breastfeed and to breastfeed the longest. The sharpest decline occurs during the early postpartum weeks. Minority women and young women tend to breastfeed for the shortest duration. Factors having the greatest impact on duration include hospital practices, obstetrical procedures, health professional contact, social support, and formula supplementation. Insufficient milk is the most common reason given for stopping breastfeeding. In addition, women stop in order to avoid breastfeeding in public and to return to work. Most women in this country follow a pattern of mixed feedings from the very beginning. Policy implications from the current research involve health professionals, hospitals, and workplaces. Further research recommendations are discussed.

BACKGROUND

Concepts about infant feeding have changed enormously over the last 50 years. Technological advances, feminism, and changing family structures have altered our practices. Nationwide studies before 1966 showed a steady decline, to a low of 18%, in the incidence of breastfeeding (1). In recent years there has been a noticeable increase in breastfeeding among some population groups. By 1983 the reported nationwide incidence had reached 61% shortly after delivery (2). Because of the newly discovered nutritional and immunological benefits of breastmilk, and the associated psychological benefits, breastfeeding is now recognized by the medical profession as the preferred method of infant feeding until 6 months of age (3). Briggs offers an excellent

196

review of current advances in knowledge about breastfeeding in Volume 1 of the *Nutrition Update* series (4).

Despite this increase in knowledge and incidence, many women encounter unanticipated obstacles and opt for formula feeding within 2 weeks of delivery (5). This chapter examines recent research on social and cultural factors that influence women to stop breastfeeding in the early postpartum period. Through a greater understanding of the social and cultural determinants of breastfeeding, health professionals can promote it more effectively.

CULTURAL FRAMEWORK

Due to the near absence of breastfeeding in our society until recently, the traditional cultural framework for breastfeeding has been virtually dissolved. Now, nursing mothers are faced with creating a new cultural framework for breastfeeding and are empirically testing its parameters.

Anne Oakley (6), an English sociologist, in her research on motherhood, contends that childbirth exists at the juncture between nature and culture. This notion can be extended to breastfeeding. Breastfeeding is a biological process dependent on the proper physiological functioning of both the mother and the infant. Although this process is created by nature, it must be learned. In the case of breastfeeding, both mother and child need to learn the techniques of breastfeeding and to adapt to one another in order to create a rhythmical milk flow. The breastfeeding process is highly sensitive to a variety of factors. Milk letdown can easily be influenced by social, psychological, environmental, and physiological variables (7). These factors are likewise part of a net of cultural practices that can either promote or inhibit lactation. Despite its natural processes, for many women lactation cannot succeed in the absence of a culturally supportive environment.

WHO BREASTFEEDS?

Demographic studies offer some clues to how the sociocultural framework around breastfeeding has changed and what factors have affected it. Studies have shown that the incidence of breastfeeding is correlated with regional variations, socioeconomic status, educational level, age, and parity (8–11). The highest incidence of breastfeeding is in the Mountain and Pacific states (12). Middle- and upper-class women led the trend away from breastfeeding and are now leading the trend back to breastfeeding. In a 1979 report for the Department of Health, Education and Welfare, Hirschman and Hendershot found that poor women who gave birth before 1960 were more likely to breastfeed than were their wealthier counterparts. However, if they gave birth after 1960, they were less likely to breastfeed (10). High educational level is also significantly correlated with a high incidence of breastfeeding. Even among low-income women, those who have attained a higher educational level tend to breastfeed (13,14). Racial and ethnic differences have also been studied. The decline in breastfeeding occurred in all groups, but the decline for black women since 1970 has been the greatest (10,15). A recent study of a community along the U.S.—Mexican border showed that the Anglo population followed the national trend in increasing breastfeeding, while the Hispanic population in this community demonstrated a decline (16). Samuels found in a heterogeneous population delivering in a health maintenance organization in Oakland, California in 1980 that over 80% of the white women breastfed; 60% of the Hispanic women breastfed; and 50% of the black women breastfed (17). A nationwide survey in 1983 found that 32% of black women and 54% of Hispanic women breastfed (2). Other researchers have found that racial differences persist even when controlling for education and parity (15).

DURATION OF BREASTFEEDING

Recent studies have shown that despite an increase in the breastfeeding rate at hospital discharge, there is a rapid decline during the postpartum period. In 1983, nationwide incidence data showed a breastfeeding rate at hospital discharge of 61% (2). At 4 months postpartum the rate was 35%. Samuels found in a California population that 58% of the breastfeeding women stopped by 4 months postpartum (17). In Western European countries the trends are similar. West, in Scotland, found that 41% stopped by 4 months, and Sjolin, in Sweden, found that 86% stopped by 4 months (18,19). Verkasalo, in Finland, found that although the incidence of breastfeeding increased between 1962 and 1972, the drop-off rate after hospital discharge was the same in both years (20). Several studies have shown that the sharpest decline in breastfeeding occurs during the first two weeks (12,17,18).

The duration of breastfeeding differs markedly among the different nations represented in the World Health Organization (WHO) Collaborative Study on Breastfeeding (21). In all nine nations represented, the duration of breastfeeding was associated with socioeconomic background. In the urban economically advantaged population, the breastfeeding prevalence at six months was never higher than 50%; whereas in the rural population 85% of the mothers were still breastfeeding at six months postpartum.

FACTORS INFLUENCING THE DURATION OF BREASTFEEDING

Studies on the duration of breastfeeding have found that those women who breastfeed the longest tend to be white, middle class, and well-educated (12,17,22). Samuels (17) found that the duration of breastfeeding was influenced by race, age, and receiving supplementary formula in the hospital. White women nursed longer than minority women. Older women nursed longer than younger women, and those women who allowed their infants to have formula while in the hospital weaned early.

Hospital practices have an important influence on the duration of breastfeeding. Medical complications and various obstetric procedures associated with delivery, such as labor induction, forceps delivery, and Cesarean section, are associated with a lower incidence of breastfeeding (23,24). Palmer et al. (25), in a study of 1356 primiparas in London, found that induction of labor and assisted delivery were significantly associated with lower breastfeeding rates. Suckling and skin-to-skin contact immediately following delivery were critical factors influencing the duration of breastfeeding. In a controlled study, de Chatean et al. (26) showed that this early contact prolonged breastfeeding by 2½ months. Sosa et al. (23) found that early infant contact extends the duration of breastfeeding. Those mothers who have rooming-in also tend to breastfeed longer (25–28). In this country, hospital practices, in general, have become more supportive of breastfeeding through the practices of natural childbirth, nursing on the delivery table, and rooming-in.

Health professionals also have an important impact on lactation. Hospitals offering programs to encourage breastfeeding tend to report a higher incidence at discharge than those with no program (28–30). Support from the hospital nursing staff influences the success of breastfeeding, although the information offered is conflicting (27). Lawrence (31), in a survey of over 1200 physicians and nurses, found that one-third of the respondents said they did not initiate a discussion of breastfeeding with their patients. Samuels found in a qualitative study of 74 breastfeeding women that none of these women indicated that any type of health professional had influenced their decision to nurse (17).

Lately attention around the world has been focused on whether the use of infant formula acts as an obstacle to both initiating and following through with breastfeeding (14,19,26,32,33). Bergevin et al. (32), in a randomized controlled clinical trial in Montreal, found that mothers randomly given formula samples in the hospital were less likely to be breastfeeding at one month and more likely to have introduced formula by two months than those mothers who received no formula in the hospital. In 1981, in response to worldwide concern over the increased substitution of formula for breastmilk and simultaneous increases in infant morbidity in developing countries, the World Health Organization passed the "International Code of Marketing of Breastmilk Substitutes," to help regulate the use of infant formula in the third world (34).

WHY WOMEN STOP BREASTFEEDING

Beyond these demographic variables and events occurring in the hospital, few studies have investigated factors during the post-hospital lactation period that predict early cessation. However, examinations of some reasons given for early cessation provide insight into potential obstacles to breastfeeding.

Cole, in a study of breastfeeding women in a Boston suburb in 1977, reports the three most common reasons given for stopping breastfeeding are: not enough milk, feeling tired, and pediatrician's recommendations (35). In a study of 239 women, West found that those women who stopped breastfeeding before 6 weeks did so because of inadequate milk, frequent feedings, fatigue, and painful nipples (18). In a 1975 prospective study conducted by the British Department of Health and Social Security, the most frequently mentioned reason for stopping breastfeeding was insufficient milk. In a 1977 Canadian study, 58% of 1039 women breastfed, but 30% stopped before 6 weeks postpartum. The most common reasons for stopping included insufficient milk, the baby nursing too often, presence of other people, cracked nipples, engorgement, and fatigue (36). Of the 840 breastfeeding mothers in a New Zealand study, 434 failed to reach their intended duration of breastfeeding. Most (81%) had stopped before 3 months, primarily because they believed their milk supply was inadequate (37). In a retrospective study conducted in Sweden, the most commonly reported reason for stopping early was "milk drying up" (19). In the WHO collaborative breastfeeding study, the most frequent reason given for stopping breastfeeding in all of the study nations, irrespective of the child's age, was insufficiency of milk (21). Samuels (17) found in a prospective study that the most common reasons for early cessation were insufficient milk, returning to work, refusing the breast, baby preferring the bottle, and weaning too early. While insufficient milk was the most common reason for stopping in the early postpartum weeks, returning to work was most common by 4 months postpartum. At the time of delivery, both concern over milk supply and plans to return to work were predictive of early cessation of breastfeeding.

Gussler and Briesemeister (38) conclude in their anthropological study of the "insufficient milk syndrome" that the "perception of insufficient milk results from general lack of knowledge about the composition of human milk and the natural and best pattern and mode of delivery." In contrast to traditional societies, where the mother and infant are in continual contact, modern society has placed distance between the nursing couple, separating the mother and the infant in the hospital, putting the infant on a feeding schedule, and waiting until the baby cries before nursing, thereby reducing the number of feedings per day.

In addition, cultural mores stand in the way and make it uncomfortable for modern women to breastfeed in public. Peters, in Seattle, found that 81% of the women studied introduced supplementary formula, primarily in order to be able to leave the house (39). This early use of formula often contributes to early cessation of breastfeeding, while the later introduction of formula tends to complement breastfeeding (17). Mixed feeding is the predominant infant feeding pattern that most women adopt; consequently, there are very few exclusively breastfed infants in this country (17,39).

Many studies emphasize the importance of support in the early postpartum period as an essential ingredient for success. The primary difference between women who stopped early and those who continued seems to be related to the availability and utilization of support systems and supportive services (27,35,36,40,41). Starling et al. found that, after hospital discharge, the mothers who had received support and encouragement to breastfeed from husbands, physicians, nurses, mothers, mothers-in-law, or La Leche League, had a significantly higher rate of success in breastfeeding (37).

Employment is also a frequent reason given for formula supplementation, since it provides additional flexibility by allowing the mother to leave her baby for longer intervals (17). However, many women stop nursing because of employment (17,42). Until the recent upsurge in breastfeeding, most breastfeeding women were privileged and did not work, lived in rural areas, or were poor and had no work (10). As more women join the labor force, this issue of working and nursing becomes more critical. Several states (Alaska, California, Hawaii, New Jersey, New York, and Rhode Island) provide an automatic 6-week paid disability leave for all employed women at a fraction of their full salary (42). Some workplaces provide longer maternity leaves, but none offer remuneration or job security during this time, forcing women to return to work before breastfeeding is well established. Other nations—France, Sweden, Japan and Israel—allow nursing breaks and remunerate women on maternity leave (42). Only two countries out of the nine study nations in the WHO Collaborative Breastfeeding Study, Sweden and Hungary, provided universal coverage for maternity leave and benefits (21).

BUILDING A CULTURAL FRAMEWORK

Ultimately, the decision to breastfeed is an individual choice and is certainly no reflection on the competency of a mother. However, this process does not occur in a social vacuum and is dependent on a number of socio-cultural variables. The absence of cultural supports may cause undue frustration and conflict for many women. The absence of abundant role models demonstrating appropriate breastfeeding etiquette and behavior leaves women confused. The absence of agreed-upon meanings leaves women feeling uncomfortable and stigmatized. As more women choose to breastfeed, there is more consensus on appropriate behavior; however, there are still serious cultural conflicts.

These cultural conflicts present important policy implications for our social system. First, health professionals need to be more sensitive to the social and cultural context for breastfeeding so they can realistically promote and support breastfeeding. Second, hospitals need to continue to change their policies to encourage breastfeeding effectively and discourage unnecessary early formula supplementation. Third, workplaces need to adopt policies that will support working mothers by allowing them extended, paid maternity leaves, nursing breaks while on the job, and/or on-the-job child care. And finally, our social customs need to adapt to the breastfeeding mother as the norm. Without all of these changes, the effective promotion of breastfeeding is unrealistic, and ultimately breastfeeding women remain outside the cultural milieu of our society. Health professionals and the society at large can help make breastfeeding easier and more feasible for more women.

RECOMMENDATIONS FOR FUTURE RESEARCH

More research is needed on barriers to breastfeeding. The following recommendations for future research have emanated from the literature (2,17,28). First, more research is needed on the effect of socioeconomic factors on breastfeeding, in order to characterize the obstacles to breastfeeding for low-income women and to study the impact of breastfeeding on the health status of infants in low-income families. Second, research is needed on hospital practices that influence breastfeeding. These include the effect of early formula supplementation, formula discharge kits, early mother-infant contact, and breastfeeding with common maternal and/or infant complications. Third, studies are needed on frequent postpartum obstacles. Nursing and employment, fertility regulation and lactation, gradual and delayed postpartum weight loss, and reduction of sexual response among lactating women are common postpartum concerns in need of further investigation. Finally, more research is needed on cross-cultural practices that will characterize breastfeeding beliefs and practices among recent immigrant populations and within different racial and ethnic groups in this country.

REFERENCES

1. H. F. Meyer, Breastfeeding in the United States: Report of a 1966 national survey with comparable 1946 and 1956 data. *Clin. Pediatr.* 7, 12, 708–715 (1968).
2. Proceedings from the Surgeon General's Workshop on Breastfeeding and Human Lactation, June 11–12, 1984, Rochester, New York. (Publ. No. HRS–D–MC–84–2) U.S. Government Printing Office, Washington, D.C., 1984.
3. American Academy of Pediatrics. Breastfeeding. *Pediatrics* 62(4), 591 (1978).
4. C. A. Briggs, Recent developments in infant feeding and nutrition. J. Weininger and G. M. Briggs, eds., *Nutrition Update*, Volume 1, Wiley, New York, 1983, p. 228.
5. P. D. Magnus and S. Galindo, The paucity of breastfeeding in an urban clinic population. *Am. J. Pub. Health* 70, 75 (1980).
6. A. Oakley, *Women Confined: Towards a Sociology of Childbirth.* Schocken Books, New York, 1980.
7. N. Newton and M. Newton, Psychological aspects of lactation. *New Eng. J. Med.* 277, 1179 (1967).
8. K. Bain, The incidence of breastfeeding in hospitals in the United States. *Pediatrics* 2, 313 (1948).
9. W. D. Robertson, Breastfeeding practices—some indication of regional variations. *Am. J. Pub. Health* 51 (7), 1035–1042 (1961).
10. C. Hirschman and G. E. Hendershot, Trends in breastfeeding among American mothers. *Vital and Health Statistics* (Series 3), Hyattsville, Maryland, November 1979.
11. D. K. Rassin, J. C. Richardson, T. Baranowski, P. R. Nader, N. Guenther, D. E. Bee, and J. P. Brown, Incidence of breastfeeding in a low socioeconomic group of mothers in the United States: Ethnic patterns. *Pediatrics* 73 (2), 132–137 (1984).
12. G. A. Martinez and J. P. Nalezienski, 1980 update: The recent trend in breastfeeding. *Pediatrics* 67 (2), 260–263 (1981).

204 NUTRITION UPDATE

13. M.T. Segeer, C.E. Gibbs, and E.A. Young, Attitudes about breastfeeding in a group of Mexican-American primigravidas. *Tex. Med.* 75, 78–80 (1979).
14. J. Mohrer, Breast and bottle feeding in an inner-city community: An assessment of perception and practices. *Med. Anthropol.* **Winter,** 125–145 (1979).
15. (Reported by) K. Fetterly and B. Graubard, Racial and educational factors associated with breastfeeding—United States, 1969 and 1980. *Morbid. Mortal. Weekly Rep.* 33, 153–154 (1984).
16. J.C. Smith, C.G. Mitango, C.W. Warren, R.W. Rochat, and S.L. Huffman, Trends in the incidence of breastfeeding for Hispanics of Mexican origin and Anglos on the U.S.-Mexican border. *Am. J. Pub. Health* 72 (1), 59–61 (1982).
17. S.E. Samuels, *Socio-Cultural Obstacles to Breastfeeding in an American Community,* Doctoral Dissertation, University of California, Berkeley, 1982.
18. C.P. West, Factors influencing the duration of breastfeeding. *J. Biosocial Sci.* 12, 325–331 (1980).
19. S. Sjolin, Y. Hofvander, and C. Hillervik, Factors related to early termination of breastfeeding: A retrospective study in Sweden. *Acta Paed. Scan.* 66, 505–511 (1977).
20. M. Verkasalo, Recent trends in breastfeeding in Southern Finland. *Acta Paed. Scan.* 69, 89–91 (1980).
21. World Health Organization, WHO Collaborative Study on Breastfeeding. Geneva, 1981.
22. D.L. Young, P.D. Mennell, M. Leung, and J. Hall, Breastfeeding: Prevalence and influencing factors. *Can. J. Pub. Health* 72, 323–330 (1981).
23. R. Sosa, J.H. Kennell, M. Klaus, and J.J Urrutia, The effect of early mother-infant contact on breastfeeding, infection, and growth. In *Breastfeeding and the Mother,* CIBA Foundation Symposium 45, Amsterdam, 1976.
24. S. Mackey and P.A. Fried, Infant breast and bottle feeding practices: Some related factors and attitudes. *Can. J. Pub. Health* 64, 780–785 (1974).
25. S.R. Palmer, A. Avery, and R. Taylor, The influence of obstetric procedures and social and cultural factors on breastfeeding rates at discharge from hospital. *J. Epid. Commun. Health* 33, 248–252 (1979).
26. P. deChateau, H. Holenberg, K. Jakobsson, and J.A. Winberg, A study of factors promoting and inhibiting lactation. *Dev. Med. Child Neur.* 19, 575–584 (1977).
27. J. Martin, *Breastfeeding.* Department of Health and Social Security, Office of Population Censuses and Surveys, London, HMSO, 1978.
28. B. Winikoff and E.C. Baer, The obstetrician's opportunity: Translating "breast is best" from theory to practice. *Am. J. Obstet. Gyn.* 138 (1), 105–117 (1980).

29. P. Verronen, J. K. Visakorpi, A. Lammi, S. Saarikoski, and T. Tamminen, Promotion of breastfeeding: Effect on neonates of change of feeding routine at a maternity unit. *Acta Paed. Scan.* **69**, 279–282 (1980).
30. K. Sloper, L. McKean, and J. D. Baum, Increasing breastfeeding in a community. *Arch. Dis. Childhood* **52**, 700–702 (1977).
31. R. A. Lawrence, Practices and attitudes toward breastfeeding among medical professionals. *Pediatrics* **70** (6), 912–920 (1982).
32. Y. Bergevin, C. Dougherty, and M. Kramer, Do infant formula samples shorten the duration of breastfeeding? *Lancet* **1**, 1148–1151 (1983).
33. A. J. Blackwell and L. Salisbury, Administrative petition to relieve the health hazards of promotion of infant formulas in the U.S. *Birth and the Family Journal* **8**, 4 (1981).
34. 34th World Health Assembly. International code of marketing of breastmilk substitutes. Resolution of the World Health Assembly, WHA 34.22, May 21, 1981.
35. J. P. Cole, Breastfeeding in the Boston suburbs in relation to personal social factors. *Clin. Pediatr.* **16**, 13–20 (1977).
36. J. E. Bergerman, E. D. Misskey, and D. A. Thompson, An overview of breastfeeding practices in three Saskatchewan health regions. *J. Can. Diet. Assoc.* **40** (3), 236–240 (1979).
37. J. Starling, D. M. Fergusson, L. J. Jorwood, and B. Taylor, Breastfeeding success and failure. *Aust. Paed. J.* **15**, 271–274 (1979).
38. J. D. Gussler and L. H. Briesmeister, The insufficient milk syndrome: A biocultural explanation. *Med. Anthropol.* **4** (2), 3–24 (1980).
39. D. C. Peters and B. Worthington-Roberts, Infant feeding practices of middle class breastfeeding and formula feeding mothers. *Birth* **9** (2), 91–96 (1982).
40. D. Raphael, *The Tender Gift: Breastfeeding.* Schocken Books, New York, 1976.
41. American Academy of Pediatrics. The promotion of breastfeeding. *Pediatrics* **69** (5), 654–661 (1982).
42. E. F. P. Jelliffe, Breastfeeding and the working woman: Bending the rules. In *Lactation, Fertility, and the Working Woman.* Proceeding of the Joint PPF/IUNS Conference, Bellagio, Italy, 1977. International Planned Parenthood Federation, London, 1979.

11
Maternal Nutrition, Fertility, and Reproductive Performance in the Preindustrialized World

BARBARA A. UNDERWOOD, Ph.D.
National Eye Institute
National Institutes of Health
Bethesda, Maryland

Address correspondence to Barbara A. Underwood, National Eye Institute, National Institutes of Health, Bethesda, Maryland 20205.

ABSTRACT

Improving the quality of life for poor families in preindustrialized nations depends upon successful family planning programs implemented concurrent with successful economic and social development programs. Success on these two fronts holds the potential for breaking the link between population growth and malnutrition among the poor within this century. Improvement in the reproductive performance of fertile women is pivotal to success. This chapter discusses issues surrounding the fertility consequences of improved maternal nutrition. Improved nutrition during pregnancy is likely to lessen maternal and perinatal mortality and, during lactation, to favor successful breastfeeding. A discussion is presented as to how, in deprived conditions, breastfeeding with the timely introduction of other foods, appropriately prepared and fed to complement breast milk, should prolong birth intervals through reduced infant mortality and lengthened periods of postpartum infertility. Evidence is also presented that indicates that improved maternal nutrition during lactation under some circumstances may hasten postpartum fertility return. The modernization and industrialization of currently preindustrialized societies and the increasing economic burden of poor families is anticipated to create such circumstances. Appropriate natural and artificial contraceptive strategies that are available to protect poor lactating women who choose to limit their fertility are discussed. A plea is made for strategies to be considered as programs and policies are developed and implemented in the critical years ahead in which we strive to meet the World Health Organization goal of "health for all" by the year 2000.

INTRODUCTION

The burgeoning and increasingly malnourished populations of preindustrialized nations continue to be of grave concern to the people of all lands and a nearly insurmountable challenge/obstacle to the World Health Organization's goal of "health for all" by the year 2000.

Only if the chain linking population growth to malnutrition is broken and the rate of increase on both fronts is slowed will it be possible to achieve this goal.

In theory, there are several approaches that could be used to intervene among the impoverished of the world in order to break the link. These include: accelerating utilization of fertility control measures, improving significantly the social and economic conditions of people at risk, and making improvements in the nutritional status of endangered populations. Economic conditions throughout the world do not look promising for an immediate improvement in economic and social conditions for the majority of the world's poor. Improvements in nutritional states are also unlikely in view of the fact that government-subsidized nutrition programs for poor fertile women are hard-pressed to compete successfully for the limited resources available for development programs generally. Although it has been demonstrated that in most industrialized nations economic and social development are followed after a lag period by a decline in the rate of population growth, there are those who would now argue, based on limited empirical data, that future improvement in the nutritional status of poor women will increase their fertility and exacerbate the problem. Indeed, there is ample evidence of physiologic relationships between fertility and *extreme* undernutrition. In extreme undernutrition, such as occurs during famines, self-induced chronic food restriction (anorexia nervosa), or secondary to disease states or heavy physical exercise, ovulation may cease or become irregular until the situation is relieved. Less clear, however, is whether mild or marginal undernutrition, the condition of most poor women in the preindustrialized world, has a direct physiologic effect on fertility.

Bongaarts (1) contends that marginal maternal malnutrition is of minimal significance in fecundity, apart from its direct or indirect effects on breastfeeding capacity and/or patterns. This topic was recently reviewed in detail by McCann et al. (2). Yet, there continue to be reports that associate an earlier postpartum return of fertility among marginally malnourished women whose nutritional status is improved but who reportedly do not alter breastfeeding practices. These findings, if validated, coupled with those showing a decline in breastfeeding and alterations in breastfeeding patterns among the poor of the preindustrialized world that are coincident with modernization and urbanization, have significant implications for policy and planning of both nutrition and fertility control programs.

DIMENSIONS OF THE PROBLEM

Of the total world population, 24% are women of reproductive age and 72% of these (about 730 million) reside in preindustrialized areas (3). Unfortunately, data on the nutrition and health status of mothers in these areas are available from only a few countries.

A realistic picture of the situation can be obtained, however, from the limited mortality data which is available in most parts of the world. Maternal mortality rates viewed globally suggest an overall decline in recent years, but this is little cause for celebration since the baseline situation may vary 30- to 200-fold between the best and worst situations. For example, the estimated *global* maternal mortality rate for 1977 was 348 per 100,000 live births (4), with rates of 1,000 or more per 100,000 live births reported for some parts of Africa and Afghanistan (5) and among some age groups within poor countries (3). These estimates exclude maternal deaths associated with abortions and stillbirths. Some maintain that the disparity in maternal mortality rates may be related to differing nutritional levels, although precise data to document this among defined populations are incomplete, and the reliability of criteria used for diagnosis of the malnutrition level is often questionable.

Maternal morbidity rates can also be used to fill in the picture of the nutritional and health status of mothers in preindustrialized countries, although data from these areas are incomplete. There is evidence that morbidity rates are elevated and that infections during gestation predispose the mother to poor pregnancy outcomes, including low-birth-weight infants. Infections during lactation also may have an adverse effect on the mother's ability to nurse and to completely carry out child care and other responsibilities. Inadequate mothering may then contribute to the poor infant growth rate and high first-year mortality common to preindustrialized areas. The implication is clear: Improved maternal nutrition could enhance survival rates of fertile women and their infants, thereby exacerbating the population problem unless direct or indirect fertility control measures are taken concurrently.

Maternal malnutrition and health in the latter period of gestation and throughout the first year are thought to relate most to infant survival. It is possible, therefore, to use perinatal and infant mortality rates (6) to gain insight into the significance of maternal nutrition in fertility and reproductive performance. Perinatal mortality includes fetal deaths after the 28th week of gestation and through the first week of life. In the preindustrialized world, deaths during this period are closely linked to **poor antenatal and obstetric care as well as to shortened birth intervals** (high parity) among women 20 years of age and under (7). Presumably this reflects, in part, poor nutritional status of the mother prior to conception and during gestation. Congenital anomalies, most of which are probably not related to nutrition, also contribute significantly to perinatal mortality (6).

A well-recognized and frequent consequence of inadequate maternal nutrition, as measured by poor weight gain during gestation, is an underweight infant. Although many factors may contribute to the birth of infants weighing less than 2500 g, maternal malnutrition, ill health, and the ecology of socioeconomic deprivation are the most common causes in the preindustrialized world. A review, reported by the World Health Organization (WHO) (8), of 80 studies in 90 countries revealed that in the Western industrialized world the incidence of low birth weight is 7–8%, a large proportion of which is associated with premature deliveries. In comparison, the incidence in less industrialized areas ranges from 11% in Latin America, to 15% in Africa, and to 31% in middle South Asia (20% for Asia as a whole).

Maternal nutrition and fertility in preindustrialized countries are influenced by infant health and survival beyond the perinatal period. In non-contracepting, breastfeeding societies these factors can determine, for example, the length of time between births. Among the world's poor, infant survival is a function of infant feeding practices, which includes not only what is fed but also the relative hygienic conditions under which feeding takes place. Infant feeding practices are influenced by the availability of money, but they are also influenced by the level of education and social awareness of the mother, as shown by Mamarbachi et al. (9). Poor hygienic feeding practices affect the health of both breastfed and bottlefed infants, although poor personal hygiene and sanitation have a relatively greater impact on those bottlefed. The early death of a breastfed infant obviously terminates breastfeeding, and frequent maternal or infant morbidity affects breastfeeding patterns. Whenever such changes in the norm occur, they have consequences for fertility return. When the return to fertility is early, and when contraception is not successfully practiced, the birth interval is frequently shortened, thereby decreasing the time available for restoration of maternal nutrient reserves. A new pregnancy superimposed on an undernourished woman increases the likelihood of another cycle of poor reproductive performance.

From available demographic and epidemiologic data, there is little doubt that maternal nutritional status is linked to the level of reproductive performance. The challenge has been to identify the risk factors associated with poor performance, how they are reflected in measurable physiological parameters, and the threshold levels at which they begin to have a significant adverse effect.

FECUNDITY, FERTILITY, AND NUTRITIONAL STATUS

Fecundity

The capacity to reproduce, or fecundity, sets the upper limit to fertility or actual reproductive performance. It is determined by both the span of years between menarche and menopause and the regularity of ovulation within that period. A conception, of course, temporarily interrupts the regularity of ovulation.

In some countries, over the last century the span of fertile years has increased as a consequence of a decline in the age of menarche. This has occurred concurrent with improved social and economic development. For example, in Scandinavia, in the 1800s, 16 years was the average age of menarche whereas it is about 13 years today (10). The age of menopause, on the other hand, appears to have remained relatively unchanged at 44–50 years (11). The earlier age of menarche is attributed by some to improved nutritional status, since the declining trends have occurred coincident with a rise in the mean body size of children for a given age, with evidence of an improved diet and with rising affluence. Others, however, are less certain of the causal relationship to nutrition under marginal conditions, since other concomitants of affluence may influence both body size and fertility (12). In any case, because of the possible linkage of fecundity to nutritional status, some argue that a demographic effect can be anticipated to parallel advances in per capita socioeconomic conditions. They urge that this be offset by intensive efforts to reach young girls and increase their understanding of family planning matters. Two points should be made, however. First, Menken and Bongaarts (13) predict little demographic impact globally from slight changes in the span of fertile years, and second, in most instances a decline in birth rates has occurred in parallel with, but lagging shortly behind, socioeconomic development, although there are exceptions reported (14). Thus, this suggests that non-physiologic factors are as (or more) significant than physiologic ones as determinants of birth rates.

Fertility

Fertility is a measure of actual reproductive performance. It is influenced by a myriad of behavioral factors, in addition to physiological ones. The behavioral factors are likely of greater importance in **determining the number and length of reproductive intervals where**

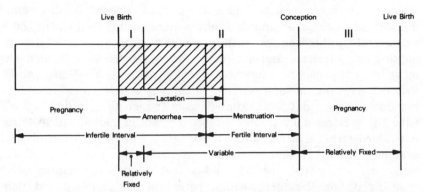

Figure 1. Conceptualization of the components of a normal birth interval. Period I is a relatively fixed infertile period following a birth. Period II among lactating women is composed of an amenorrheic interval of variable length determined in part by breastfeeding patterns and perhaps maternal nutrition, and a menstruating fertile interval. Frequency of sexual activity and contraceptive practices influence the length of the fertile period to conception. Period III is gestational interval, normally relatively fixed in length but shortened by abortions.

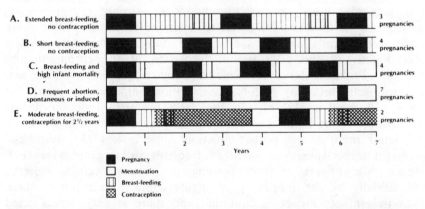

Figure 2. Different patterns of breastfeeding and contraception and their impact on fertility. (Adapted with permission from reference 2.)

marginal undernutrition prevails than are physiologic ones. Figure 1 conceptualizes the components of the birth interval as consisting of three periods. The first is an intractile period of postpartum infertility usually lasting four to nine weeks and virtually uninfluenced by nutritional state. The second is the period from the time the tissue integrity has been reestablished and the next conception; this period includes a lactational amenorrheic and a menstruating component and is significantly influenced by maternal nutrition both directly through physiologic correlates and indirectly through behavioral factors, the most important of which are breastfeeding patterns. The third period, that of gestation, is least variable in length and least influenced by marginal states of nutrition. Alterations in the length of period two will have the greatest demographic effects. Factors in addition to maternal nutritional status that can affect the length of this period include, for example, infant feeding patterns that influence the span of the lactational amenorrhea period, and sexual activity and contraceptive practices during the menstruating period of the lactating and non-lactating intervals. How variations in these factors could in theory influence fertility are illustrated in Figure 2 (2). The following discussion focuses on recent information regarding how these factors and maternal nutrition influence segment II of the interbirth interval.

Infant Feeding Patterns: Full Breastfeeding

Evidence has been available for many years that breastfeeding lengthens the period of postpartum amenorrhea. The underlying physiological control mechanism, however, is only recently being understood. It involves the pituitary hormone prolactin. Prolactin, in addition to stimulating milk synthesis, is thought to depress ovulation and directly or indirectly inhibit formation of the corpus luteum (15,16). Prolactin levels are elevated by nipple stimulation, and hyperprolactinemia may prolong the lactational amenorrhea period for up to 18 months (17,18). In the early postpartum period, tactile stimulation of the nipple causes a spiking in serum prolactin levels; in the latter months, the post-stimulation surge is less (15) but basal prolactin levels remain elevated by frequent suckling episodes (19). Hence, the effects of breastfeeding on fertility can be altered substantially by the frequency of nipple contact. In cultures where maternal—infant contact is continual and there is easy, unrestricted access to the breast as is typical in rural Bangladesh (20), India (21), among the traditional !Kung hunter—gatherers (22), and some sections of Africa (18,23,24), lactational amenorrhea may last 12—18 months or longer and birth intervals be prolonged for 24—36 months or more. In comparison, amenorrhea may be as short as 6—8 weeks where a neonatal death has occurred or where separation of the dyad is customary and hence limits the frequency of contact stimulation.

Intensity of suckling also has been suggested as a factor that modifies breastmilk production. Presumably, this would be mediated through the prolactin response (15), but this has not been fully documented. It is the rationale Whitehead et al. (25) used to explain their observation of an association between birth weight of Gambian infants and the volume of milk their mothers produced at the second month of lactation. They reasoned that heavier newborns sucked more intensely during the formative period when controls over lactation capacity were being set. The magnitude of the post-stimulation prolactin spike is assumed to be greater, at least in the early postpartum period, following a more intense suck pressure. This assumption needs to be verified, but advancements in this area are limited by the lack of precise tools for measuring suck pressures that do not interfere with the natural feeding process (26). This technological limitation has led to use of the time spent at the breast as a surrogate for the intensity measurement. The relationship is that the more intense the suck, the shorter the duration on the breast that is needed to deplete the milk reservoir (15). Lucas et al. (27) using a cross-sectional study design, showed that healthy 6-day-old infants in Britain obtained about 50% of their total intake per feeding from the breast in the first 2 minutes and up to 90% at 4 minutes. Unfortunately, they did not concurrently measure maternal prolactin levels.

Because of the implications for intervention programs, studies are needed of the associations between suckling intensity and duration among babies of varying birth weights, and maternal prolactin levels and milk output. There are trade-offs that should be considered. For healthy normal-weight infants, the shorter the suckling time to fulfill nutritional needs, the greater the chance for an earlier maternal ovulatory breakthrough, although perhaps she will have a greater milk production capacity. In some circumstances, means of facilitating more frequent contact stimulation might be the appropriate intervention, while in others, artificial contraceptives may be more appropriate. Infants born weak, of low birth weight, or who become weakened later, who may suckle longer but less intensely, may require a different intervention strategy. In these cases, perhaps a means of increasing the intensity of nipple stimulation through adjunct measures may be needed to induce an adequate prolactin response for maximizing both milk production and the antiovulatory effect (28). Among marginally nourished societies, a better understanding of these basic relationships is central to the issues of increasing the prospects for infant survival and catch-up growth (28).

Infant Feeding Patterns: Partial Breastfeeding

Virtually all infants of poor mothers in the preindustrialized world need food to complement breastmilk by 6 months of age and frequently by 3 to 4 months; occasionally, depending on individual circumstances, there is need at an even earlier age. The evidence for this has been reviewed recently (29). Although there are conflicting and non-conclusive reports from the preindustrial world (23,30), most studies indicate that the lactational amenorrhea period ends shortly after complementary food is introduced (31−33). This presents a dilemma: How do poor mothers who want to regulate their fertility adequately meet the nutritional needs of the nursling for complementary food while maintaining the full contraceptive effects of breastfeeding? Can this be achieved by altering the pattern of offering the complementary food relative to the breast? Are different breastfeeding patterns the reason for the apparently conflicting reports from different societies?

The importance of obtaining answers to these questions is illustrated by studies comparing women from industrialized and preindustrialized societies. McNeilly et al. (16) showed that among well-nourished lactating women in Scotland, food complementation was associated with a rapid decrease in the total duration of suckling, a decline in the maternal serum prolactin levels, and a resumption of follicular development. Serum prolactin levels remained significantly above the normal level at which ovulation occurs in this population (>400 mU/liter, [34]) for at least 7 months postpartum, as long as breastfeeding continued. The return of fertility among these well-nourished women was attributed to a decrease in suckling duration, presumably a consequence of reduction of the infant's dependence on breastmilk for meeting his full nutritional need. Unfortunately, the investigators did not report how complementary food was fed relative to breastfeeding, that is, whether the infant was first allowed to suckle to satisfaction, then the food complement used to top off the feeding, or vice versa.

In contrast to the findings from Scotland, Vis and Hennart (23), among some marginally nourished rural African tribes where there is no dietary substitute for mother's milk, found that semi-solid local food introduced as a breast milk complement as early as 15−21 days postpartum did not influence maternal prolactin levels. Indeed, mean serum prolactin levels among these women who suckle their infants frequently, and during the night, remained above the threshold where ovulation reoccurs in this population (<800 mU/liter) up to approximately 15 months (35). In the African culture, the mother/infant dyad is in almost continuous contact for at least 18 months postpartum, and the complementary food, which is frequently pre-chewed, is given while maintaining natural on-demand access to the breast (17,23). Is the difference between these two cultures in basal prolactin levels attributable to duration of nipple contact only, or is the amount and perhaps the manner in which complementary food is fed important? Can this account for the individual variations reported in fertility return among similarly undernourished women of preindustrialized societies? If so, this behavior may be amenable to simple educational interventions readily incorporated into nutrition, family planning and other maternal and child health (MCH) programs, and into institutional practices. In theory, providing the breast first should take greatest advantage of the infant's hunger and thirst drives to encourage vigorous suckling; this could be muted if the complementary food were first provided. Alternately, the thirst drive may be paramount in encouraging suckling. If true, then first feeding semi-solid food (lesser water content than breastmilk) could enhance this need, hence, subsequently encourage a vigorous suck, though perhaps of shorter duration, at the breast. Research is urgently needed to clarify how patterns of breast/complementary feeding modulate maternal circulating prolactin levels and as a consequence, fertility and possibly sustained milk output (36).

Sexual Activity During Lactation

Sexual activity during lactation has been limited by tradition in many cultures (37). Among those cultures, prolonged breastfeeding, therefore, has effectively contributed to maintenance of long birth intervals, at least of 2 years or more. These traditions, especially those that prescribe strict abstinence, appear to be breaking down and, in addition, the length of the breastfeeding period is declining. These trends are occurring particularly as the educational level of women increases, as urbanization and modernization occur, and as the availability of artificial contraceptive alternatives improves (38,39). A shortened birth interval is noted for many young urbanized African women as a consequence of these factors (40,41).

Contraceptive Practices

Acceptance of family planning through natural and/or artificial means has been variable in the preindustrial world. In general, a direct relationship exists between levels of education and family planning acceptance. Hence, those with higher levels of formal education, usually associated with a higher level of affluence, are more prone to find means of controlling their fertility than are the less educated.

Frequently they utilize artificial contraception such as oral or injectable contraceptives, intrauterine devices (IUDs), or physical barriers (2) in preference to dependence on natural fertility control, such as prolonged, full breastfeeding or coitus interruptus (30). However, in some cultures there is resistance toward prolonged, uninterrupted use of the most effective contraceptives (42). Natural contraception other than full, frequent breastfeeding is notoriously unreliable, particularly among poorly educated women (43). Experience in Bangladesh has demonstrated that intensive family planning, health service programs that offer a wide variety of contraceptive methods adaptable to individual requirements, can influence contraceptive utilization across age groups and socioeconomic levels (44). The importance of integrated family planning and MCH activities to breastfeeding practices is illustrated by experiences in Malaysia (39,45). Malaysian women were more likely to breastfeed where there were integrated services. They did tend to wean their infants earlier where artificial contraceptives were available as alternatives to prolonged breastfeeding. Nonetheless, their newborn infants had received the early biosocial and biomedical benefits of breastfeeding. The most cost-effective intervention where female illiteracy prevails to achieve a synergistic beneficial effect on both fertility trends and infant feeding practices may be an upgrading in the general educational level of women. Certainly, modernization will continue to penetrate traditional societies. Failure to prepare women to adapt appropriately to these influences by making informed choices that maximize benefits for their family circumstances could have serious negative consequences both for individual infants and their families (9) and for population control (14,46).

NUTRITIONAL STATUS DURING LACTATION AND AMENORRHEA

Will an improved nutritional status of lactating women through diet cause an earlier return of fertility when breastfeeding duration and frequency are unchanged? This important question has enormous relevance for policy and programs in the preindustrialized world. There are strong pressures on governments to provide feeding programs to poor pregnant and lactating women on the assumption that by "feeding the mother you are feeding the child." It is assumed that better maternal nutrition will improve infant survival and milk production capacity. Hence, this would enable women to meet their surviving infant's nutritional needs through breastfeeding for a longer period, with the potential for a prolonged period of lactational amenorrhea if the latter benefit is not nullified by ovulation occurring sooner when the plane of maternal nutrition is raised. To resolve the question of the role of the plane of maternal nutrition on fertility, two types of studies are available for analysis: (1) cross-sectional studies in which maternal anthropometric measures are used to classify nutritional levels and retrospective histories to establish fertility measures, and (2) prospective studies in which fertility measures are directly ascertained and, in some cases, food supplements are provided.

Two cross-sectional studies reported from Bangladesh found no evidence from maternal anthropometric nutritional indicators of a significant association with either the duration of the postpartum amenorrhea interval or of the menstruating interval prior to the next conception (47,48). Neither of these studies controlled for breastfeeding patterns or duration. Contrasting findings are reported from Africa and India. Caraël (49) reported a cross-sectional retrospective study in Zaire among the Havu in the eastern highlands and the Ntomba and Tembo in the tropical equatorial forest area that showed a correlation between anthropometric indices of nutritional status and length of the postpartum amenorrhea period. He provided additional evidence that differences in maternal dietary factors accounted for the differences in the length of the postpartum amenorrhea interval. Prema et al. (50), in a cross-sectional retrospective study among Indian women, noted a progressive fall in the duration of lactational amenorrhea with increasing maternal body weight. Again, however, neither the African or Indian studies can be considered more than suggestive that maternal nutritional level influenced the timing of fertility return since infant feeding patterns were not evaluated.

Few prospective studies are reported. Among those that provided food supplements, Delgado et al. (51) reported a negative association in a calculated nutritional status index and the length of postpartum amenorrhea among Guatemalan Indian women who had received measured food supplement during pregnancy. A negative association was found between caloric intake during pregnancy and the length of postpartum amenorrhea. Similar associations, not always statistically significant, were found between other nutritional indicators and the amenorrheic period. The duration of lactation over a 24-month postpartum period, however, was the primary determinant of the amenorrheic period; caloric intake accounted for approximately a 1- to 2-month shortening of the period between the low- and high-intake groups. These findings are confounded since some infants as well as their mothers were supplemented and there was no control for changes that might have occurred in suckling patterns. Similar reservations in interpretation apply to the otherwise carefully controlled studies of Chavez et al. (52), who reported a decline by 7 months in the postpartum amenorrheic period among a small group of Mexican mothers provided food supplements during pregnancy and lactation. In subsequent studies on women from this same population, Chavez is reported to have shown that when the *infants* were not supplemented, the mean amenorrheic interval was no different whether or not the *mothers* were supplemented [cited in Bongaarts (1)].

Further analysis, reported by Delgado et al. (53), of the data from Guatemala seems to support the hypothesis that maternal nutritional status indirectly influences fertility by determining the availability of breastmilk, hence, the frequency, duration, and intensity of suckling. These investigators assume that these parameters, in turn, influence prolactin and other hormonal balances associated with ovarian activity and development of the corpus luteum, hence, the postpartum infertility interval (16,54). That milk output is decreased by serious maternal energy deficit is supported by studies where marked seasonal variations in food availability occur (17,55). However, supplementing the diet of the marginally malnourished mother does not unequivocally lead to an increased milk volume (56), whereas it does lead to lowered circulating level of prolactin (57) and a substantially shortened period of postpartum amenorrhea (58). Studies in the Gambia (56) and Zaire (59) note that these changes in prolactin levels are responsive to maternal nutritional adequacy independent of changes in the frequency of breastfeeding. This conclusion argues for a substantial independent effect of maternal nutritional status on the length of the lactational amenorrhea period and is in contrast to the conclusion reached by Delgado (52), Bongaarts (1), and Chowdhury (47).

Note should be taken that supplementation of mothers in the Gambia to improve their nutritional plane resulted in subjective evidence of benefit to their life quality. The food supplementation program was reported to be very popular because the recipients believed they had more energy for carrying out their responsibilities (46). These subjective reports are reminiscent of similar benefits noted in supplementation programs for marginally nourished young children who become more "naughty" after food supplementation but among whom differences could not be measured through anthropometric indices.

Regardless of mechanism, the implication of the studies reviewed is that in breastfeeding populations living under conditions of chronic marginal malnutrition, an improvement in maternal diet is likely to hasten the decline in circulating levels of prolactin and lead to an earlier fertility return irrespective of infant feeding patterns. If the latter is also altered, fertility may return even sooner. Among non-contracepting societies, the positive health benefits of improved nutrition could be offset by a shortened birth interval. Yet, there are obvious quality-of-life benefits to the mother from improving her level of nutrition, and the means are available for controlling fertility while lactation continues.

POLICY AND PROGRAM IMPLICATIONS OF IMPROVED MATERNAL NUTRITION FOR REPRODUCTIVE PERFORMANCE

The physiological and life-quality benefits of an improved nutritional status for reproducing women and their families argue both on a personal and population level for programs to improve the diet of those even marginally inadequate. However, because of their potential personal consequences and demographic implications, these programs need to be coupled with those that provide fertility protection to women who choose to control their reproductive performance. The most desired approach to fertility control is to take maximal advantage of the antifertility effects of natural full breastfeeding described earlier in this chapter. This approach also provides all the socio-medical benefits to the infant that have been reviewed exhaustively elsewhere. The first three postpartum months are the most critical for providing these benefits to the offspring. This period is characterized for most women, even those marginally nourished, by the ability to produce milk of adequate quantity and quality for their infant's nutritional needs. Full natural breastfeeding for a 3-month period would likely extend the infecundable interval by 1 to 2 months. Adjunct contraceptive measures, then, are unlikely to be needed on a population basis before the fifth month postpartum. Studies have shown the importance of avoiding double coverage of fertility, that is, introducing artificial contraception while lactational infertility remains effective. Too-early use of artificial contraception when unnecessary is associated with early discontinuation. This may leave a woman vulnerable at a time when the infertility effect of breastfeeding has waned and artificial contraception is needed (44,46). The guiding principle for policy and programs, therefore, should be to protect at least this 3-month period postpartum, insofar as the local and individual circumstances permit.

In many cases, circumstances permit the period of full natural breastfeeding to be extended beyond 3 months, and this will extend antifertility and health benefits to the mother and infant. But, for a growing number of poor women in urban and rural areas, economic necessity is forcing changes in lifestyles that are not compatible with extended periods in which the traditional pattern of natural breastfeeding can continue. Many of these women must resume their responsibilities for family welfare, often necessitating entry or reentry into the formal or informal labor market. They are able to continue to breastfeed, but not with the natural frequency necessary to sustain the antiovulatory effects of hyperprolactinemia. Often their infants need a food complement to the breastmilk they can provide. For these women, policies and programs that provide ready access to adjunct contraceptive measures appropriate to their cultural heritage and lifestyle and which favor continued lactation are needed. What these appropriate alternative contraceptives are and when they should be introduced was recently summarized in the report of a workshop sponsored by the WHO and the National Academy of Sciences (46). Hormonal contraceptives are not to be encouraged during the period when lactation continues because of the effect of even small amounts (30 μg) of estrogen on the volume of milk produced, the duration of lactation, and the possibility of their transmission to the infant in breastmilk. (Note that there is no clear evidence that the small amount transmitted to nursing infants is harmful.) Progesterone-only hormonal contraceptives do not appear to affect milk volume. Contraception by sterilization or by physical barriers such as condoms, foams, or spermicidal agents does not interfere with lactation. IUDs are appropriate in the latter postpartum months, but there is a higher risk of expulsion or perforation in the earlier postpartum months. Once lactation has ceased, hormonal contraceptives can be safely used.

There is much emphasis on policies and programs for the promotion of breastfeeding in both industrialized and preindustrialized societies. This focus of attention on the importance of breastfeeding has reversed the declining trend, irrespective of economic status, in several industrialized societies. The effectiveness of such programs in slowing the declining trend in preindustrialized societies is less clear. The forced change in lifestyles for many poor women, as noted earlier, is causing them to depend more and more on an early food complement to the diet of their infant. They frequently have neither time to prepare an appropriate complementary food from local resources or the money to buy one available commercially. These realities, in part beyond their control, leave these women vulnerable to continued poor reproductive performance and place their families in high-risk categories for poor health and poor social outcomes.

SUMMARY

Many arguments can be made for improving the nutritional status of women in their reproductive years. The foregoing review of current knowledge of the potential fertility consequences, whether through direct or indirect mechanisms, highlights the importance of integrating nutrition, MCH, and family planning programs. Only then will there be assurance that the overall consequences will likely improve the quality of life. To achieve this, some issues for which answers are urgently needed include a better understanding of how complementary food can be provided in a way that does not depress lactation performance, maximizes the antifertility effects of breastfeeding, and provides maximum protection and nutritional benefit to the infant. Without doubt, appropriate policies and programs for the preindustrialized world to support these concepts will involve improvement in environmental sanitation, in the availability of potable water, and in the education of women, not only in nutrition and personal hygiene, but generally to assist them in better utilizing the emerging resources available to them within their particular environmental and economic context.

REFERENCES

1. J. Bongaarts, Does malnutrition affect fecundity? A summary of evidence. *Science* **208**, 564 (1980).

2. M. F. McCann, L. S. Liskin, P. T. Piotrow, W. Rinehart, and G. Fox, Breast-feeding, fertility and family planning. *Population Reports*, Vol. IX, No. 5, Part 1, Series J, No. 24, The Johns Hopkins University, 1981.

3. World Health Organization. Sixth Report on the World Health Situation 1973–1977. Part I: Global analysis. WHO, Geneva, 1980.

4. R. W. Rochat, Maternal mortality in the United States of America. *World Health Stat. Q.* **34**, 2 (1981).

5. T. Dyson, Infant, child and maternal mortality and associated conditions of health in the greater Kabul region of Afghanistan. *World Health Stat. Q.* **34**, 14 (1981).

6. A. Ashworth, International differences in infant mortality and the impact of malnutrition: A review. *Hum. Nutr: Clin. Nutr.* **36C**, 7 (1982).

7. H. Goldstein, Factors related to birth weight and perinatal mortality. *Br. Med. Bull.* **37**, 259 (1981).

8. Division of Family Health, World Health Organization, The incidence of low birth weight—A critical review of available information. *World Health Stat. Q.* **33**, 197 (1980).

9. D. Mamarbachi, P. L. Pellett, H. M. Basha, and F. Djani, Observations on nutritional marasmus in a newly rich nation. *Ecol. Food Nutr.* **9**, 43 (1980).

10. P. B. Eveleth and J. M. Tanner, eds., *Worldwide Variation in Human Growth*, Cambridge University Press, London, 1976.

11. H. Leridon, ed., *Human Fertility*, University of Chicago Press, Chicago, 1977.

12. L. Zacharias and R. J. Wurtman, Age at menarche: Genetics and environmental influences. *New Engl. J. Med.* **280**, 868 (1969).

13. J. Menken and J. Bongaarts, Reproductive models in the study of nutrition–fertility interrelationships. In W. H. Mosely, ed., *Nutrition and Human Reproduction*, Plenum, New York, 1978, pp. 261–311.

14. A. Romaniuk, Increase in natural fertility during the early stages of modernization: Canadian Indians case study. *Demography* **18**, 157 (1981).

15. J. E. Tyson and A. Perez, The maintenance of infecundity in postpartum women. In W. H. Mosely, ed., *Nutrition and Human Reproduction*, Plenum, New York, 1978, pp. 11–27.

16. A. S. McNeilly, P. W. Howie, and M. J. Houston, Relationship of feeding patterns, prolactin, and resumption of ovulation postpartum. In G. I. Zutuchni, M. J. Labbok, and J. J. Sciarra, eds., *Research Frontiers in Fertility Regulation*, Harper & Row, New York, 1980, pp. 102–116.

17. Ph. Hennart and H. L. Vis, Breast-feeding and post partum amenorrhoea in Central Africa. I. Milk production in rural areas. *J. Trop. Pediatr.* **26**, 177 (1980).

18. M. Caraël and J. B. Stanbury, Promotion of birth spacing in Idjwi Island, Zaire. *Stud. Fam. Plann.* **14**, 134 (1983).

19. B. A. Gross and C. J. Eastman, Prolactin secretion during prolonged lactational amenorrhoea. *Aust. N.Z. J. Obstet. Gynaec.* **19**, 95 (1979).

20. S. L. Huffman, A. K. M. A. Chowdhury, J. Chakraborty, and N. K. Simpson, Breast-feeding patterns in rural Bangladesh. *Am. J. Clin. Nutr.* **33**, 144 (1980).

21. R. Rajalakshmi, Gestation and lactation performance in relation to the plane of maternal nutrition. In H. Aebi and R. Whitehead, eds., *Maternal Nutrition During Pregnancy and Lactation*, Nestle Foundation Workshop, April 26–27, 1979 (Lausanne), Nestle Foundation Publication Series No. 1, Hans Huber Publishers, Bern, Stuttgart, Vienna (Wein): Huber, 1980, pp. 184–202.

22. M. Konner and C. Worthman, Nursing frequency, gonadal function, and birth spacing among !Kung hunter–gatherers. *Science* **207**, 788 (1980).

23. H. L. Vis and Ph. Hennart, Decline in breast-feeding: About some of its causes. *Acta. Paediatr. Belg.* **31**, 195 (1978).

24. R. J. Wenlock and R. W. Wenlock, Maternal nutrition, prolonged lactation and birth spacing in Ethiopia. *J. Biosoc. Sci.* **13**, 261 (1981).

25. R. G. Whitehead, M. G. M. Rowland, M. Hutton, A. M. Prentice, E. Muller, and A. Paul, Factors influencing lactation performance in rural Gambian mothers. *Lancet* **2**, 178 (1978).

26. R. F. Drewett and M. Woolridge, Sucking patterns of human babies on the breast. *Early Hum. Dev.* **3/4**, 315 (1979).

27. A. Lucas, P. J. Lucas, and J. D. Baum, Pattern of milk flow in breast-fed infants. *Lancet* **2**, 57 (1979).

28. V. DeSanctis, U. Vitali, G. Atti, C. Vullo, A. Sabato, and B. Bagni, Comparison of prolactin response to suckling and breast pump aspiration in lactating mothers. *Ric. Clin. Lab.* **11**, 81 (1981).

29. B. A. Underwood and Y. Hofvander, Appropriate timing for complementary feeding of the breast-fed infant. *Acta Paediatr. Scand.* [Suppl.] 1982, pp. 1–32.

30. J. Knodel, P. Kamnuansilpa, and A. Chamratrithirong, Breastfeeding in Thailand: Data from the 1981 contraceptive prevalence survey. *Stud. Fam. Plann.* **13**, 307 (1982).

31. M. F. El-Minawi and M. S. Foda, Postpartum lactation amenorrhea. *Am. J. Obstet. Gynecol.* **111**, 17 (1971).

32. H. Delgado, E. Brineman, A. Lechtig, J. Bongaarts, R. Martorell, and R. E. Klein, Effect of maternal nutritional status and infant supplementation during lactation on postpartum amenorrhea. *Am. J. Obstet. Gynecol.* **135**, 303 (1979).

33. K. Prema, A. N. Naidu, and S. Neela Kumari, Lactation and fertility. *Am. J. Clin. Nutr.* **32**, 1298 (1979).

34. P. W. Howie, A. S. McNeilly, M. J. Houston, A. Cook, and H. Boyle, Effect of supplementary food on suckling patterns and ovarian activity during lactation. *Br. Med. J.* **283**, 757 (1981).

35. P. Delvoye, P. M. Desmaegd, Uwayitu-Nyampeta, and C. Robyn, Serum prolactin, gonadotropins, and estradiol in menstruating and amenorrheic mothers during two years' lactation. *Am. J. Obstet. Gynecol.* **130**, 635 (1978).

36. K. Prema and M. Ravindranath, The effect of breastfeeding supplements on the return of fertility. *Stud. Fam. Plann.* **13**, 293 (1982).

37. J.-F. Saucier, Correlates of the long postpartum taboo: A cross-cultural study. *Curr. Anthro.* **13**, 238 (1972).

38. V. J. Hull, A study of birth interval dynamics in rural Java. In W. H. Mosely, ed., *Nutrition and Human Reproduction,* Plenum, New York, 1978, pp. 433–459.

39. J. DaVanzo and W. P. Butz, Birthspacing, fertility and family planning. Policy and program implications from the Malaysian family life survey. Rand Publication Series, R-2925-AID, Santa Monica, Cal., 90406, 1981.

40. N. Rehan and A. K. Abashiya, Breastfeeding and abstinence among Hausa women. *Stud. Fam. Plann.* **12**, 233 (1981).

41. H. J. Page and R. Lesthaeghe, eds., *Child-spacing in Tropical Africa: Traditions and Change,* Academic, London, 1981.

42. S. Bhatia, S. Becker, and Y. J. Kim, The effect on fecundity of pill acceptance during postpartum amenorrhea in rural Bangladesh. *Stud. Fam. Plann.* **13**, 200 (1982).

43. H. Zurayk, Breastfeeding and contraceptive patterns postpartum: a study in South Lebanon. *Stud. Fam. Plann.* **12**, 237 (1981).

44. S. Bhatia, Contraceptive users in rural Bangladesh: a time trend analysis. *Stud. Fam. Plann.* **14**, 20 (1983).

45. W. P. Butz, J.-P. Habicht, and J. DaVanzo, Improving infant nutrition, health, and survival. Policy and program implications from the Malaysian family life survey. Rand Publication Series, R2924-AID, Santa Monica, Cal., 90406, 1981.

46. WHO/NRC, Breastfeeding and fertility regulation: Current knowledge and programme policy implications. Report of a Workshop. *Bull. WHO* **61**, 371 (1983).

47. A. K. M. Chowdhury, Effect of maternal nutrition on fertility in rural Bangladesh. In W. H. Mosely, ed., *Nutrition and Human Reproduction*, Plenum, New York, 1978, pp. 401—410.

48. S. L. Huffman, A. K. M. Chowdhury, and W. H. Mosley, Postpartum amenorrhea: How is it affected by maternal nutritional status? *Science* **200**, 1155 (1978).

49. M. Caraël, Relations between birth intervals and nutrition in three Central Africa populations. In W. H. Mosley, ed., *Nutrition and Human Reproduction*, Plenum, New York, 1978, pp. 365—384.

50. K. Prema, A. N. Naidu, S. Neelakumari, and B. A. Ramalakshmi, Nutrition-fertility interaction in lactating women of low income groups. *Br. J. Nutr.* **45**, 461 (1981).

51. H. Delgado, Nutrition and birth interval components: The Guatemalan experiences. In W. H. Mosley, ed., *Nutrition and Human Reproduction*, Plenum, New York, 1978, pp. 385—399.

52. A. Chavez and C. Martinez, Nutrition and development of infants from poor rural areas. III. Maternal nutrition and its consequences on fertility. *Nutr. Repts. Int.* **7**, 1 (1973).

53. H. L. Delgado, R. Martorell and R. E. Klein, Nutrition, lactation, and birth interval components in rural Guatemala. *Am. J. Clin. Nutr.* **35**, 1468 (1982).

54. R. G. Whitehead, ed., Maternal Diet, Breastfeeding capacity, and lactational fertility. *Food Nutr. Bull.* [Suppl.] **6**, 1983.

55. A. A. Paul, E. M. Muller, and R. G. Whitehead, The quantitative effects of maternal dietary energy intake on pregnancy and lactation in rural Gambian women. *R. Soc. Trop. Med. Hyg.* **73**, 686 (1979).

56. A. M. Prentice, R. G. Whitehead, S. B. Roberts, A. A. Paul, M. Watkinson, A. Prentice, and A. A. Watkinson, Dietary supplementation of Gambian nursing mothers and lactational performance. *Lancet* **2**, 886 (1980).

57. P. G. Lunn, A. M. Prentice, S. Austin, and R. G. Whitehead, Influence of maternal diet on plasma-prolactin levels during lactation. *Lancet* **1**, 623 (1980).

58. P. G. Lunn, M. Watkinson, A. M. Prentice, P. Morrell, S. Austin, and R. G. Whitehead, Maternal nutrition and lactational amenorrhoea. *Lancet* **1**, 1428 (1981).

59. P. Delvoye and C. Robyn, Breast-feeding and post partum amenorrhoea in Central Africa. II. Prolactin and post partum amenorrhoea. *J. Trop. Pediatr.* **26**, 184 (1980).

Nutrition Education

12
Nutrition Education
ADVANCES IN ACCESSIBILITY AND EFFECTIVENESS

HELEN D. ULLRICH, M.A., R.D.

Nutrition Communications Associates
Berkeley, California

Address correspondence to Helen D. Ullrich, M.A., Nutrition Communications Associates, 1116 Miller Avenue, Berkeley, California 94708.

ABSTRACT

Nutrition education programs have grown more in direction and effectiveness in the past 10 years than in any previous period. This has been due partly to the expansion in nutrition intervention programs after the 1969 White House Conference on Food, Nutrition and Health. Two significant advances are the Nutrition Education and Training (NET) program in schools and the establishment of the Dietary Guidelines for Americans. The former improves access to sound nutrition information in schools. The latter is a national nutrition policy statement that expands beyond the basic four food groups as a teaching tool. New programs have been started, such as supermarket consumer programs and community-wide health education.

Nutrition education programs include a variety of motivational techniques to help the learner gain understanding of the art, science, and technology of food and nutrition and the relationship to health, disease, and the total environment in keeping with one's own lifestyle, economics, and social and cultural priorities.

Many health and education professionals are nutrition educators, but it's a small component of their job, and their training often is meager. Nutritionists are challenged to meet these needs and continue the major advances that have been made in nutrition education research and evaluation methodologies.

BACKGROUND

Nutrition education has received considerable attention in recent years. The increased knowledge and interest in nutrition have contributed to the need for more effective nutrition education programs. Traditionally, nutrition education has been issue-related. When specific issues about the nutritional well-being of individuals and the population are identified, then there is a need to educate people about these issues.

One of the early attempts at nutrition education involved teaching the homemaker how to preserve and conserve food during World War I and feeding and educating poor and hungry school children (1).

230

Today's proliferation of knowledge of the effects of the interactions of nutrients on the health and well-being of the population has given rise to controversy and variations in interpretation. The selection of food in relation to food safety, ecology, energy resources, and economics adds still another dimension of concern. Therefore, nutrition education requirements are much more sophisticated. The expectations and ability to measure success of programs have also grown in recent years.

This chapter concentrates on the period from 1974 through 1982, when the major advances were made in defining and addressing problems relating to nutrition education. This parallels the period of major national interest in the development of national policies on nutrition programs and controversies related to the state of knowledge about nutrition. Probably the two most significant accomplishments during the period were the issuance of *Nutrition and Your Health— Dietary Guidelines for Americans* (2) as a result of the cooperative efforts of federal government agencies, and the appropriation of funds to facilitate the development of a Nutrition Education and Training (NET) program in schools nationwide (3).

Perhaps the most important event to shape the direction of today's activities in nutrition education was the 1969 White House Conference on Food, Nutrition and Health (4). The pressures brought to bear by citizen groups concerned about hunger forced the scientists as well as politicians to look at nutrition issues in relation to the social and economic needs of the poor and hungry. As a result, there was major growth in programs such as food stamps, child and elderly feeding, and Head Start programs. Programs specifically extending access to nutrition education included the Food and Drug Administration (FDA) nutritional labeling and the Expanded Food and Nutrition Extension Program (EFNEP), which focused on low-income families, and eventually the NET program as a part of the National School Lunch Act.

Education of the public about the existence of hungry people in the United States in the late 1960s is an example of how a problem can be addressed and an aroused public and legislature will effect changes (5). An initial thrust of great impact on public attitude was a CBS television network documentary "Hunger in America," first aired in May of 1968. That was followed by several articles and books such as the special feature "Hunger in Our Midst" in the Charlotte, N.C., *Observer* (6) and the book by Nick Kotz, *Let Them Eat Promises— The Politics of*

Hunger in America (7). The White House Conference was a response to the public outcry about hunger.

Two evaluative bibliographies of the literature about malnutrition as it relates to children and their learning abilities summarize the research through the mid-1970s (8,9). Both reviews indicated that hungry children exhibit behavioral changes that may limit their response to learning opportunities. Chronic malnutrition has some correlations as well.

The educational approaches to combat malnutrition as they were understood in the late 1960s and early 1970s were summarized by Ullrich and Briggs (10). They indicated that when setting up a community-type program, whether on a national, state, or local level, one must assess the needs of the community, its resources, options for disseminating information, manpower available for teacher training and dissemination of knowledge, periods of human openness to change during the life span, and types of communication within the community, as well as the education resources.

There are compendia giving a historic perspective on nutrition education in the United States. An annotated bibliography on published works about methods and kinds of nutrition education from 1961 to 1972 reflects that much of what was published showed relatively isolated, small programs involving a minimum of coordination and evaluation (11). Gussow, and others who contributed to the *Teachers College Record* in 1980, review the past and give a perspective to the future needs, which must include far more than simply the study of nutrients and how they affect the body (12). Approaches to education must include where and how food is grown, processed, and available to the consumer, and the politics and policies that affect the nutritional quality of the available food.

This chapter also discusses some of the advances in evaluating the effectiveness of existing programs. Abt Associates, under contract to the USDA to evaluate the effectiveness of NET programs, prepared a review of nutrition education programs and research (13). The review was limited to education components related to NET: teacher and school food service personnel training, education from preschool through secondary school with a conceptual framework for individual nutrition, and the state of the art of nutrition education evaluation. The review points out that nutrition education is relatively undeveloped. There are few identifiable theoretical approaches; furthermore, approaches to behavioral change are not well defined, and there is little recognition of a multitude of factors besides nutrition knowledge which influence behavior.

WHAT IS NUTRITION EDUCATION?

The terms nutrition education and nutrition information are sometimes used interchangeably. People need to have information in order to build a body of knowledge from which to take action to assure their nutritional well-being. The kind and quality of information are components of nutrition education. However, it should not be considered sufficient to ensure a successful program that will bring about a desired change. It may take a variety of motivational techniques to change habits. A definition I have used and found to be acceptable to the educational community is: "Nutrition education is the process which enables individuals to gain understanding and skills necessary to protect and improve (originally "promote") their nutritional well-being through their food choices" (14). In today's world, with the proliferation of information and increased controversy about nutrition and health issues, it becomes increasingly difficult to have an understanding of one's own nutritional needs. This understanding would be drawn from knowledge of nutrition as it relates to health and disease; the art, science, and technology of food and nutrition; and how they relate to the total environment as well as one's own lifestyle, economics, and social and cultural priorities. The development of skills to make economically satisfying choices and select and prepare foods in tasteful combinations are all a part of the total process. This means that the process is ongoing throughout a lifetime. An adequate overall nutrition education program should provide ways for individuals to interact with new findings, ideas, and concepts constantly. The professional is challenged to develop many ways to disseminate information as well as to use a variety of learning techniques.

Contento (15) has stated that:

> in trying to satisfy the goal of producing healthy people while meeting the needs of the learner or consumer in implementing that goal, the field of nutrition education has been in conflict over the extent to which it needs to relate to its disciplinary roots in the field of .biochemistry. As a consequence, nutrition educators have sometimes rather narrowly focused their attention on teaching people how to apply nutrition science principles to food selection, failing to take into sufficient account the rapid changes in the food supply or the consequent changed educational needs of consumers. The field has also not drawn as much as it might from the disciplines of anthropology, sociology, psychology and economics—to name just a few—in elucidating why we eat what we do, how food and its use affect the well-being of individuals and society or how we might

design nutrition education strategies that are more appropriate to the task at hand.

The National Nutrition Consortium issued a statement on Nutrition Education Policy in June 1980 (16). The following are the points that they consider to make up a sound policy:

1. As part of a concern for the total health and well-being of the individual, nutrition education should be incorporated into all educational levels from preschool to university, including graduate and professional schooling.
2. The home is the basic learning center for food and nutrition knowledge, attitudes, and practices; thus, in order to ensure continuity in the educational process, efforts should be directed toward improved programs for adult education.
3. Nutrition education programs should be conducted or supervised by professionals who have had scientific training in nutrition through accredited institutions.
4. The content of nutrition education should be based on scientific evidence and, where appropriate, should present both sides of a controversial issue.
5. All nutrition efforts should include an evaluation component assessing attitudinal, cognitive, and/or behavioral change.
6. Adequate funding for continuing research in nutrition education must be made available from both public and private sources.
7. In order to implement the activities proposed in points 1–6, there must be coordinated efforts on the part of all those involved in nutrition education including various agencies of the federal government, industry, nutrition and home economics educators, state departments of health and education, universities and professional schools, teacher education programs, and recognized organizations committed to nutrition and nutrition education.

NUTRITION EDUCATION POLICY DEVELOPMENT

The most active time in the development of nutrition education policy was between 1974 and 1979. The buildup of interest was the result of legislative committees taking on this charge in the Senate and the House. In June of 1974, the Senate Select Committee on Nutrition and Human Needs held a series of hearings titled "National Nutrition Policy Study." The panel reports and public hearings were designed to follow up federal actions after the 1969 White House Conference on Food, Nutrition and Health. While there was specific emphasis on nutrition education issues addressed in the Consumer and Nutrition Panel through a subpanel on Popular Nutrition Education, the panels on Special Groups, Food Availability, and Health all made reference to the increased need for nutrition education (17). Shortly after the hearings, Senator George McGovern introduced the "National Nutrition Education Act of 1974" (18). In doing so, he indicated that at the hearings "We heard over and over again the refrain 'You must feed people' but food is meaningless without nutrition education."

The bill, in its original form, was addressed to the then Office of Education. It provided for technical assistance, teacher training, planning and organization, and curriculum development; a Nutrition Education Coordinator in each state; a National Nutrition Education Resource Center for training, collection, and creation of curricula and other materials; and evaluation of state-level programs. It asked for 75 million dollars. In October of 1977, after the demise of the Senate Select Committee, Congress passed the Nutrition Education and Training legislation as a part of the National School Lunch Act of 1977. Funding was based on 50 cents per school child per year starting in Fiscal Year 1978 (3). This was about 28 million dollars. The funds were cut back each year until Fiscal Year 1983 funds were at the level of 5 million dollars (19). The same level was maintained in 1984. Though this program has always been plagued by limited funds, it has provided the opportunity to introduce and integrate nutrition education concepts into the school curriculum and increase the coordination of the school feeding programs with the educational program. However, without funds it may not be possible to expect a sustained effort.

The Food and Drug Administration (FDA) voluntary program on nutritional labeling was in place and functioning relatively well soon after the White House Conference. But, another area of access to information that had never been addressed to any great extent was nutritional misinformation via food advertising. In the fall of 1974, the Federal Trade Commission (FTC) introduced a proposal to regulate the kinds of nutritional claims that could be made about food. The purpose was to provide guidance for making nutritional claims in food advertising (20). In addition, in 1978 the FTC responded to concerns consumers expressed about food advertising on television programs directed to children (21). The agency proposed regulations banning all advertising to very young children and advertising of highly sugared foods to children 8 to 11 years of age and certain other ads to be balanced by nutritional and/or health disclosures funded by advertisers. In 1981, the FTC role was redefined and all progress to regulate a more balanced nutrition message in advertising ended (22). A glance at today's food advertising shows a high percentage of nutritional claims: some accurate, some misleading, and some inaccurate.

In 1976, a special committee of the Society for Nutrition Education looked at ways in which foods could be called a good source or an excellent source of certain nutrients in response to the FTC's proposed recommendations (23). While those proposals were never adopted, they remain a valid and reliable way of grouping foods to help in rating foods as poor, good, or excellent sources of specific nutrient.

The House Subcommittee on Domestic Marketing, Consumer Relations and Nutrition of the Committee on Agriculture held hearings on nutrition education for consumers in 1977 and 1978 (24,25). The committee also introduced a bill to establish a Federal Nutrition Education Council, but no action was taken. There have been several attempts to establish such a council, but the alternate solution was to establish a joint subcommittee on human nutrition research, which contained a nutrition education research component.

A multitude of studies and reports was prepared during those years. Various legislators requested reviews of government programs by the Library of Congress and the General Accounting Office (26–32). A study was carried out by The President's Reorganization Project in 1978 (33). The Department of Health and Human Services (DHHS) published reports on health and disease prevention in 1979 which included nutrition education needs (34,35). The flurry of activity culminated in a National Conference on Nutrition Education in the Fall of 1979 (36). There was an effort to engender broad involvement of federal, state, and local agencies, private industry, academia, health professionals, and consumers in addressing the issues related to the needs in nutrition education and recommending policy.

In 1982, the Joint Subcommittee on Human Nutrition Research issued a report which identified the departments within agencies where there were research activities with a nutrition education and training component (37). It is of interest to note that in the National Institutes of Health (NIH) budget for Fiscal Year 1980, $7.6 million, or 5.5 percent of the $139-million program for biomedical and behavioral nutrition research was devoted to nutrition education research. This research was carried out as a component of prevention and intervention programs and clinical trials. The Centers for Disease Control (CDC) devoted $630,000 to special state-level nutrition activities. The Department of Agriculture indicated that in Fiscal Year 1980, which was the peak year for nutrition funding, $107 million was allocated for nutrition education of the public.

During 1981 and 1982, efforts were made to form the Network for Better Nutrition (NBN), an organization that would have had broadly based representation from government, consumers, the food industry, and professionals. The intent was that the NBN would spearhead activities related to increasing public awareness and understanding about nutrition. However, government support and financial backing were not adequate to get it underway.

WHO ARE NUTRITION EDUCATORS?

In the broadest sense, anyone who is communicating information about food and nutrition might be considered a nutrition educator. There should be standards of qualification for persons who carry out these activities. The problem is that many professionals and nonprofessionals who disseminate the information have had little or no formalized training in nutritional sciences. As a result, the quality of nutrition education is very mixed, ranging from in-depth, balanced review of the state of knowledge about nutrition to folklore and blatantly false claims. Additionally, there are few people beyond the academic setting who are full-time nutrition educators. Instead, "nutrition educator" activity is often a component of a broader job description, such as dietitian, home economist, consumer affairs specialist, health, science, or physical education teacher, physician, dentist, nurse, food editor, and retail store clerk.

Some progress has been made in defining roles and training. For example, in a 1982 report on public health nutrition, education is identified as a major or intermediate role for all public health nutrition personnel except the dietetic technicians in nutrition care (38). Guidelines for education and training are given.

In 1978, the Society for Nutrition Education published recommendations on functions and qualifications of the nutrition education specialist in formalized education, grades K–12 (39). Those standards have been useful in establishing qualifications for nutrition education coordinators in state and local NET programs. In 1981, an SNE "Scopes and Priorities of Nutrition Education Committee" was established to identify competencies common to all nutrition specialty areas and those which differentiate the nutrition education specialist from other specialty areas (40).

In a USDA survey of consumer opinions taken in 1980, 38% of respondents indicated that the doctor/dentist/nurse was the most influential source of information influencing household dietary change. Only 5% considered the dietitian/nutritionist or public health educator as the primary source (41). In 1982, when a group of physicians was asked which health promoting behaviors they perceived as "very important" for the average person, 70% listed "avoid excess calories" and 58% listed "eat a balanced diet." And, 47% routinely asked patients about diet (42).

The health professional is the most effective promoter of behavioral changes made by the public, and there have been some efforts to increase the amount of pre-service and in-service training. Fiscal Year 1980 was a peak year for federal expenditures in this area. In that year, $6.8 million was spent on training, and 90% of that was for the health professional (37). In 1982, Dr. James Long urged health professionals to assess and reduce the barriers to the practice of nutritionally sound medicine (43). One problem he identified was physicians not taking the time to learn what must be learned to be well informed about nutrition.

On the other hand, there are diploma mills that continue to perpetuate myths and misinformation about nutrition by making it easy to get a bachelor's and/or graduate degrees by correspondence. Virginia Aronson described the ease with which a "degree" with a diploma as a nutritionist could be obtained by correspondence from Bernadean University and noted that the textbooks for the course contained inaccurate and faddist information (44).

The only nutrition professional who has certification is the registered dietitian. All other terminology, such as nutritionist or nutrition educator, has not been agreed upon within the professional nutrition groups. Thus, the public cannot be expected to understand the differences in capabilities and knowledge of those who communicate nutrition information in various forms and by various methods.

The challenge for the professionally trained nutritionist who is functioning at some level as an educator is to find ways to work cooperatively with those who need to have specific kinds of information in order to be effective nutrition educators. The nurse, elementary teacher, senior citizen volunteer, fitness counselor, the store clerk— each has specific nutrition knowledge needs. Shannon found that while adequate training of the teachers is important, a positive attitude and commitment are also necessary (45).

TECHNIQUES AND TOOLS OF NUTRITION EDUCATION

Just as the public interest in nutrition has increased in recent years, the kinds of techniques and programs to respond have increased. For example, at the Society for Nutrition Education's 1974 Annual Meeting there were 24 papers presented that described innovative programs and related research (46). At SNE's 1982 Annual Meeting, 120 papers and poster presentations were given (47). While the number of books received for review by the *Journal of Nutrition Education* (approximately 150) did not increase over the same span of years, 104 educational materials were listed in 1974, and 203 were listed in 1982. The materials include only those available for purchase. There are many more available for use in state and local programs that are not submitted for review in the professional journals.

As mentioned earlier, one of the most significant accomplishments during this period was the development of *Nutrition and Health: Dietary Guidelines for Americans* jointly published by USDA and DHHS in 1980 (2). Dwyer has analyzed events and policies involved in establishing those guidelines (48). From the nutrition educator's point of view, the guidelines provided recommendations that were not a part of the four food groups of the Daily Food Guide. For a long time, nutritional scientists had published research data related to cholesterol, fat, carbohydrate, and sodium in the diet. However, The Food and Nutrition Board of the National Academy of Sciences, which was responsible for establishing the Recommended Dietary Allowances (RDA) in 1980, did not make specific recommendations for those components of the diet in relation to various age groupings (49). Nutrition educators felt they were without sufficient guidance to make recommendations to the public. While the nutrition educator can observe and identify problems related to specific dietary practices, it is the authoritative groups such as the Food and Nutrition Board which are looked to for a review of the state of knowledge and research and to establish recommendations on dietary needs.

The Dietary Guidelines on cholesterol, fat, sugar, and sodium are general in nature as opposed to the *U.S. Dietary Goals* published by the Senate Select Committee on Nutrition and Human Needs (50). Nevertheless, the guidelines provide a national statement on which educational programs can be built.

Nutrition education researchers have evaluated food guidance tools and several alternate plans have been suggested (51–53). Guthrie found that self-selected diets of a group of adults which fulfilled the four food groups recommendations contained at least 80% of the RDAs for all nutrients (54). The question remains whether that is an acceptable goal; the problem is whether it is possible to devise a simple food guidance tool that is universal enough to accomodate all types of eating patterns. Can the same guide accommodate persons who prefer a minimum variety of foods eaten in two or three meals a day as well as those who choose foods like pizza, casserole dishes, and easily available fast foods eaten haphazardly throughout the day? Can the same guide be used for a relatively high-animal-protein and a vegetarian diet?

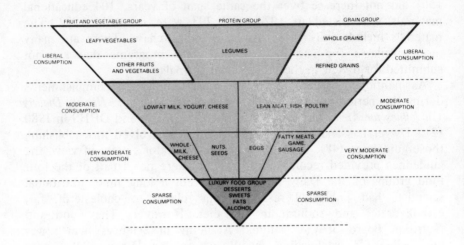

Figure 1. Inverse pyramid food guide (from reference 52).

Dodds suggests a more universal grouping of foods that reflects the way foods grow (51). Called The Handy Five, its groups are: 1) Flesh around seeds (fruit); 2) leaves, stalks, roots, and flowers (vegetables); 3) seeds or grasses (grains); 4) seeds in pods (nuts and legumes); and 5) animal products (dairy, eggs, and meat). Pennington has developed a four-layered reverse pyramid with a broad top strata including foods for liberal consumption and narrowing to a bottom strata of sparse consumption foods (52). This grouping encourages selection of nutrient-dense foods and discourages consumption of foods high in fat, cholesterol, sugar, and salt (Figure 1). Any plan devised to incorporate the current knowledge of nutrition requires considerable translation in order to personalize it for individual use.

Nutrition educators should look to new ways to expand the audiences they reach. Guthrie points up ways by which the nutrition educator's spheres of influence can be expanded by teaming up with other professionals such as teachers, health educators, media specialists, peer educators such as weight control program directors, and food marketing specialists (55). One of the most recent techniques having phenomenal growth is the use of the computer. Numerous diet analysis, food consumption, menu planning, and food buying programs have been developed. Nutrition information should be integrated into software and games programs now being used in the home. Cable TV and home video tapes could provide still another means to reach large audiences.

At the 1969 White House Conference, a conceptual framework for nutrition education was recommended (4). In 1980, a revision of the framework was published by a committee of the Society for Nutrition Education (56). The revised concepts are a series of statements which are considered by the committee to be important ideas about nutrition in general, food and its handling, nutrients and dietary components, nutritional and physical fitness, food selection, and national and international policies. These concepts are useful in organizing objectives for a nutrition education curriculum.

The specific techniques of using different kinds of educational media such as print, audiovisual, and games have met with various degrees of success with a variety of audiences. Publications such as the *Journal of Nutrition Education* and the *Journal of the American Dietetic Association* contain many articles that provide examples of methods and techniques from individual counseling to national mass media programs for consumers, patients, school children, and professionals. The major change during this period was use of measurable goals and objectives for nutrition education programs with evaluation carried out on the effectiveness of the technique under the conditions in which it was used.

ACCESSIBILITY

The federal government has been the major financial supporter of the dissemination of information used in nutrition education programs at the state and local levels. There was a modest growth in the mid to late 1970s in nutrition education funds as a part of federally funded nutrition intervention programs. It was estimated in 1976 that USDA and DHEW supported roughly $70 million worth of nutrition education activities (57). In 1980, USDA alone allocated $107 million for nutrition education of the public (37). However, there were drastic budget cuts since 1980 and in 1983 USDA is expected to discontinue providing any publications free of charge through the Consumer Information Center (58).

Federal programs have never attained their potential outreach. A U.S. General Accounting Office study in 1978 found that USDA's Extension Food and Nutrition Program reached only 2% of its intended audience, and the Expanded Food and Nutrition Education Program barely 20% (27). As far as DHEW programs were concerned, Head Start reached 15%, nutrition programs for the elderly 23%, and consumer adult education programs only 2% of the target populations. There were almost 400 publications on food and nutrition available from these two agencies; the one with the highest distribution was a publication on holiday meals which stressed food safety (3,000,000 copies). Next was *Food Is More Than Just Something to Eat* with a distribution of about 1,500,000.

Mass media has increased the consumer's access to information. The largest source of information about food is advertising. In 1981, the 18 major food companies listed in the top 100 advertisers in the United States spent $1.257 billion for television time (network and spot) and $277 million for space in newspapers and general circulation magazines (59). The majority of such advertising is for foods that are highly-processed and contain large amounts of sugar and fat (60). A sizable portion of the advertising for sugared cereals, soft drinks, and candy is aimed at children via the TV shows they watch. Efforts have been made to produce public service announcements (PSAs) to put the nutritional message into perspective. Some PSAs promoting fruits and vegetables such as tomatoes, citrus, grapes, and so forth have been produced and distributed by organizations such the Produce Marketing Association, United Fresh Fruit and Vegetable Association, and other marketing groups for specific foods. Some Federal and state agencies have produced TV spots on subjects such as dental health, heart disease, and so on. However, PSAs do not receive the frequency of airing that paid advertising gets. Manoff recommended at the 1979 National Conference on Nutrition Education that there be a public policy requiring a fixed share of TV and radio time be mandated to health and nutrition education (61).

There is increased access to information in retail food stores. Several supermarket chains have initiated educational programs through their consumer affairs departments. Giant Foods, under a contract with DHHS–NIH, developed a storewide program called Foods for Health (37). As a part of the program, 3,000,000 copies of a publication "The Eater's Almanac" were distributed. Groups like the American Heart Association have adopted the program and will be distributing it throughout the country. Safeway and Kroger are two other major food store chains that have recently initiated active consumer education programs.

The popular press has exhibited a strong interest in nutrition. Several newspapers and women's magazines like *Redbook* and *Woman's Day* provide the nutrient content of their recipes. Parham et al. looked at weight control as portrayed in 33 issues of 22 popular magazines (62). They found for the most part that the articles measured up very well on the ideas considered to be important in a presentation on weight control. However, it was pointed out that one cannot assume accuracy for every article. Each needs to be evaluated individually. Hudnall reviewed a range of nutrition articles in 19 major magazines over the last 10 years (63). Those which were given ratings of 90% or better include *Redbook*, *Reader's Digest*, and *Good Housekeeping.* At the bottom of the list with less than 3% were *Harper's Bazaar*, *Organic Gardening*, and *Prevention.*

Access to nutrition education materials for grades K—12 educational programs has been greatly increased because of the federal NET monies. Most states either developed their own materials or established a listing of curriculum materials for use in classrooms. The National Dairy Council developed curriculum materials for use in preschool through secondary education. Many local dairy councils disseminated the programs through local teacher-training programs. Those materials are the most widely used throughout the country.

Probably the largest privately funded, statewide multifaceted nutrition education project was carried out by The Pennsylvania State University through a grant from The Nutrition Foundation and Heinz Foundation. On a pilot project research basis, it contained aspects of health professional and teacher training, curriculum development, public education programs, and continuous access to information through a nutrition education resource center.

The concept of resource centers at national, state, and local levels has grown and, while there is no definitive study as yet of the roles and functions of such centers, they generally provide information and services for professionals and the public. The services may range from answering questions on a one-to-one basis to providing a newsletter and loaning materials. The USDA Food and Nutrition Information Center (FNIC) housed in the National Agricultural Library has an AGRICOLA data base of more than 20,000 citations (37). Its services are currently available only to extension and school food service personnel and certain other USDA groups.

While there appears to be a sizable expansion of available nutrition information, much of the work has been on a pilot project level; funds for printing materials have been greatly restricted, and the means to train teachers and paraprofessionals to use available materials effectively are very limited because federal funds have been curtailed since 1980.

EVALUATION

Some of the nutrition education activities carried out during the past 10 years have been effective. A USDA consumer survey in 1979 indicated that two-thirds of the households surveyed reported dietary changes for reasons of health or nutrition during the previous three years (64). More than half had been influenced by a health professional. One-third cited the media as their source of influence.

Long-term disease prevention programs, such as the Stanford Heart Disease Prevention Program and MRFIT, have studied a variety of intervention procedures that include nutrition education and have found that people can be motivated to change. The Stanford Study has shown that lasting changes can be achieved on a community level through health education (65).

Considerable progress has been made in identifying nutrition education research needs that would determine how, why, what, and when nutrition education is effective. Two government reports identified areas of priority for research: (1) to improve understanding of the factors affecting dietary practices, food consumption patterns, and their determinants, (2) to develop and refine methodologies for nutrition education and communication, (3) to improve the effectiveness and efficiency of nutrition education programs, and (4) to expand research training and manpower development in nutrition education (37,66).

Many leaders in nutrition education met three times during 1980–81 to establish directions for research (67–69). The workshops identified and discussed some of the behavioral science methodologies and theoretical frameworks which should be considered in future research. Evaluative instruments have been developed for many types of programs. A full issue of the *Journal of Nutrition Education* was devoted to the subject (70). Talmage and Rasher caution that a test which is valid and reliable for one group may not be equally so for all groups (71).

Evaluation has become a required component of most nutrition education programs. The NET program requires evaluation on an ongoing basis. One of the reasons why funding was originally approved for NET was because of the lack of evaluation of the effectiveness of the school lunch program and rising public concern about food waste. For this reason, many states have included a plate waste measurement in their NET evaluation. When the nutrition education project has been directed at consumption of specific foods, a very measurable decrease in plate waste has been repeatedly demonstrated (72).

Many of the nutrition intervention programs have suffered financial cutbacks because evaluation mechanisms were not built into the programs. Unfortunately, the results of extensive evaluation of projects started in the late 1970s were not ready when Congress started cutting social programs in 1980. As the results have become available in 1982–1983, it should help at least to stabilize the programs and reassure the taxpayers that their money was well spent.

CONCLUSIONS

It appears that the great groundswell of interest in nutrition continues in the early 1980s. Nutrition is a household word. Nutrition education now includes reaching people who have a myriad of lifestyles and addressing issues such as breastfeeding and food supply. People have begun to take control of their health by adjusting their food habits along with physical activity. The profession of those looked to for nutrition information has changed greatly. Nutritionists are now challenged to find ways to work cooperatively with other health and physical fitness professionals, teachers, food retailers, communicators, agriculturalists, and consumers, to name a few, and to assist in providing a base line of balanced nutrition information to respond to the zeal for nutrition "cures."

In the next 10 years, there will be many breakthroughs in nutritional science as it relates to the lifestyles of the people. In turn, the accessibility and effectiveness of nutrition education and nutrition educators will expand.

REFERENCES

1. E. A. Martin, Historical foundations for nutrition education research. In J. K. Brun, ed., *Nutrition Education Research Directions for the Future*, National Dairy Council, Rosemont, Ill., 1980, p. 3.
2. U.S. Department of Agriculture and U.S. Department of Health and Human Services. *Nutrition and Your Health, Dietary Guidelines for Americans*, Washington, D.C., 1980.
3. Anon., Congress passes nutrition education bill. *J. Nutr. Ed.* **9**, 168A (1977).
4. Anon. *White House Conference on Food, Nutrition and Health*, U.S. Government Printing Office, Washington, D.C., 1970.
5. H. D. Ullrich, Hunger in America and nutrition education. *J. Nutr. Ed.* **1**(1), 5 (1969).
6. *A Special Report, Hunger in Our Midst*, OEO Pamphlet 1405–6, reprinted from the Charlotte, N.C., *Observer* by the Office of Economic Opportunity, Washington, D.C., 1969.

7. N. Kotz. *Let Them Eat Promises—The Politics of Hunger in America*, Prentice-Hall, Englewood Cliffs, N.J., 1969.
8. Anon. *Relationships of Hunger and Malnutrition to Learning Ability and Behavior*, Department of Citrus, Lakeland, Fla., 1979.
9. R.Y.L. Tseng, J. Mellon, and K. Bammer, *The Relationship between Nutrition and Student Achievement, Behavior and Health— A Review of the Literature*, California State Department of Education, Sacramento, 1980.
10. H.D. Ullrich and G.M. Briggs, Education to combat malnutrition. In D.S. McLaren, ed., *Nutrition in the Community*, Wiley, London, 1976, p. 245.
11. C.S. Wilson and S. Knox, Methods and kinds of nutrition education (1961—72): A selected annotated bibliography. *J. Nutr. Ed.* 5 (Supp. 2) (1973).
12. J.D. Gussow, ed., Learning and eating: The new nutrition education. *Teachers College Record* 81, 411 (1980).
13. J.P. Nestor and J.A. Glotzer, eds. *Teaching Nutrition*, Abt Books, Cambridge, Mass., 1981.
14. H.D. Ullrich, Towards a national nutrition education policy. *J. Nutr. Ed.* 11, 60 (1979).
15. I. Contento, Thinking about nutrition education: What to teach, how to teach it, and what to measure. *Teachers College Record* 81, 421 (1980).
16. National Nutrition Consortium, Statement of nutrition education policy. *J. Nutr. Ed.* 12, 138 (1980).
17. Anon., National nutrition policy, A special report. *J. Nutr. Ed.* 6 (Insert i—viii) (1974).
18. Anon., Legislation corner. *SNE Communicator* 5(3), 14 (1974).
19. M. Mathieu, Legislative highlights. *J. Am. Diet. Assoc.* 82, 189 (1983).
20. Anon., Proposed food advertising regulations: Comment by Feb. 5, 1975. *SNE Communicator* 5(4), 4 (1974).
21. Anon., FTC issues report restricting TV advertising to children. *SNE Communicator* 9(1), 5 (1978).
22. Anon., FTC kills rule on food advertising. *CNI Weekly Report* xii(50), 7 (1982).
23. Anon. *Nutritional Claims for Food*, Society for Nutrition Education, Oakland, Cal., 1976.
24. Anon. *Nutrition Education. Hearings before the Subcommittee on Domestic Marketing, Consumer Relations, and Nutrition, 95th Congress, First Session*, Serial No. 95-Z, Part 1, U.S. Government Printing Office, Washington, D.C., 1977.
25. Anon., *Nutrition Education, National Consumer Nutrition Information Act. Hearings before the Subcomittee on Domestic Marketing, Consumer Relations, and Nutrition, 95th Congress, Second Session*, Serial No. 95-Z, Part 2. U.S. Government Printing Office, Washington, D.C., 1978.
26. Congressional Research Service, The Library of Congress. *The Role of the Federal Government in Nutrition Education.* U.S. Government Printing Office, Washington, D.C., 1977.

27. Comptroller General of the United States. *Informing the Public about Nutrition: Federal Agencies Should Do Better*, CED-78-75. U.S. Government Accounting Office, Washington, D.C., 1978.

28. Comptroller General of the United States, *Federal Human Nutrition Research Needs a Coordinated Approach to Advance Knowledge*, Vol. 1, PSAD-77-156. U.S. General Accounting Office, Washington, D.C., 1978.

29. Comptroller General of the United States. *Federal Domestic Food Assistance Programs—A Time For Assessment and Change.* CED-78-113. U.S. General Accounting Office, Washington, D.C., 1978.

30. Comptroller General of the United States. *Recommended Dietary Allowances More Research and Better Food Guides Needed,* CED-78-169. U.S. General Accounting Office, Washington, D.C., 1978.

31. Comptroller of the United States. *What Foods Should Americans Eat? Better Information Needed on Nutritional Qaulity of Foods.* CED-80-68. U.S. General Accounting Office, Washington, D.C., 1980.

32. Anon. *What Can Be Done to Improve Nutrition Education Efforts in the Schools?* GAD/CED—82—65. U.S. General Accounting Office, Washington, D.C., 1982.

33. President's Reorganization Project. *Food and Nutrition Study Final Report.* Executive Office of the President, Washington, D.C., 1978.

34. Anon. *Preventing Disease/Promoting Health.* Department of Health, Education and Welfare, Washington, D.C., 1979.

35. Surgeon General of The Public Health Service. *Healthy People,* DHEW (PHS) Publication No. 79—55071. U.S. Government Printing Office, Washington, D.C., 1979.

36. J. Dwyer, ed., National nutrition conference on nutrition education. *J. Nutr. Ed.* **12** (Supp. 1), (1980).

37. Joint Subcommittee on Human Nutrition Research. *Federally-Supported Human Nutrition Research, Training, and Education. Update for the 1980s. III. Nutrition Education Research and Professional Personnel Needs for Nutrition Education of Professionals and the Public.* National Technical Information Service, Springfield, Va., 1982.

38. M. Kaufman, ed. *Personnel in Public Health Nutrition for the 1980's.* Association of State and Territorial Health Officials Association, McLean, Va., 1982.

39. Anon., Nutrition education specialists in school systems, K—12: A position paper on functions and qualifications. *J. Nutr. Ed.* **10**, 6 (1978).

40. B. Shannon, Scope and practice of nutrition education. *SNE Communicator* **12**(3), 4 (1981).

41. J. J. Putnam and J. Weimer, Nutrition information—Consumer's views. *National Food Review* **14**, 18 (1981).

42. H. Wechsler, S. Levine, R. K. Idelson, M. Rohman, and J. O. Taylor, The physician's role in health promotion—A survey of primary-care practitioners. *New Eng. J. Med.* **308**, 97 (1983).

43. J. M. Long, III, Opening the closet door: The key is education. *J. Par. Entr. Nutr.* **6**, 280 (1982).

44. V. Aronson, Bernadean University: A nutrition diploma mill. *ACSH News & Views* 4(2), 7 (1983).
45. B. Shannon, P. Bell, E. Marbach, L. H. O'Connell, K. L. Graves, and R. F. Nicely, Jr., A K−6 nutrition curriculum evaluation−Instruction and teacher preparation. *J. Nutr. Ed.* **13**, 9 (1981).
46. Anon., Annual meeting highlights, Part 1. *SNE Communicator* 5(3), 2 (1974).
47. Anon., *SNE Abstracts: #7 Programs and Research in Nutrition Education, 1982 Abstracts.* Society for Nutrition Education, Oakland, Cal., 1982.
48. J. Dwyer, Dietary recommendations and policy implications. In J. Weininger and G. M. Briggs, eds., *Nutrition Update,* Vol. 1, Wiley, New York, 1983, p. 315.
49. Committee on Dietary Allowances, Food and Nutrition Board, National Research Council. *Recommended Dietary Allowances,* 9th ed, National Academy of Sciences, Washington, D.C., 1980.
50. S. M. Oace and H. D. Ullrich, eds., U.S. dietary goals. *J. Nutr. Ed.* **9**, 152 (1977).
51. J. M. Dodd, The handy five food guide. *J. Nutr. Ed.* **13**, 50 (1981).
52. J. A. T. Pennington, Considerations for a new food guide. *J. Nutr. Ed.* **13**, 53 (1981).
53. P. A. Lachance, A suggestion on food guides and dietary guidelines. *J. Nutr. Ed.* **13**, 56 (1981).
54. H. A. Guthrie and J. C. Scheer, Nutritional adequacy of self-selected diets that satisfy the Four Food Groups guide. *J. Nutr. Ed.* **13**, 46 (1981).
55. H. A. Guthrie, Nutrition education−Challenges and partnerships. *Food and Nutrition News* 54(1), 1 (1982).
56. Anon., SNE concepts for food and nutrition education. *J. Nutr. Ed.* **14**, 1 (1982).
57. C. E. Woteki, Building consensus for nutrition education research. *J. Nutr. Ed.* **11**, 7 (1979).
58. Anon., Consumer update. *CNI Week* **xiii**(17), 7 (1983).
59. Anon., 100 leaders' media expenditures compared in 1981. *Advertising Age* 53(38) (Sept. 9), 12 (1982).
60. A. E. Gallo and J. M. Connor, Advertising and American food consumption. *National Food Review* 19, 2 (1982).
61. R. K. Manoff, The new politics of nutrition education. *J. Nutr. Ed.* **12** (Supp. 1), 112 (1980).
62. E. S. Parham, V. L. Frigo, and A. H. Perkins, Weight control as portrayed in popular magazines. *J. Nutr. Ed.* **14**, 153 (1982).
63. M. Hudnall, ACSH survey: How popular magazines rate on nutrition. *ACSH News & Views* 3(1), 1 (1982).
64. J. L. Jones and J. Weimer, Health-related food choices. *Family Economics Review,* Science and Education Administration, U.S. Department of Agriculture, Washington, D.C., Summer 1981, p. 16.
65. S. P. Fortmann, P. T. Williams, S. B. Hulley, W. L. Haskell, and J. W.

Farquhar, Effect of health education on dietary behavior: The Stanford Three Community Study. *Am. J. Clin. Nutr.* **34**, 2030 (1981).

66. Office of Technology Assessment. *Nutrition Research Alternatives.* U.S. Government Printing Office, Washington, D.C., 1978.
67. C. M. Olson and A. H. Gillespie, eds., Proceedings of the workshop on nutrition education research. *J. Nutr. Ed.* **13** (Supp. 1), (1981).
68. Anon. *Directions for Nutrition Education Research— The Penn State Conference, A Proceedings.* The Pennsylvania State University, University Park, Pa., 1980.
69. J. Brun, ed. *Proceedings of Nutrition Education Research Conference— Strategies for Theory Building.* National Dairy Council, Rosemont, Ill., 1983.
70. S. M. Oace, ed., Perspectives on nutrition education instrumentation. *J. Nutr. Ed.* **13**, 83 (1981).
71. H. Talmage and S. P. Rasher, Validity and reliability issues in measurement instrumentation. *J. Nutr. Ed.* **13**, 83 (1981).
72. K. L. Clancy, Testimony before the Subcommittee for Nutrition, Senate Committee on Agriculture, Nutrition and Forestry, Feb. 23, 1982 (unpublished).

ADDITIONAL RECENT REFERENCES

73. Office of Disease Prevention and Health Promotion. Public Health Service implementation plans for attaining the objectives for the nation. *Public Health Reports,* Supplement to Sept.-Oct. (1983).
74. C. S. Wilson, A. Maretzki, and H. Talmage, *Profiling Nutrition Education Materials. An Instrument with Manual.* Society for Nutrition Education, Oakland, Cal., 1983.
75. B. Shannon, ed., Computers in nutrition education. *J. Nutr. Ed.* **16**, entire June 1984 issue.
76. R. K. Manoff, New directions in nutrition education. *J. Food and Nutr.* **40**, 60 (1984).

13
Television's Role in Nutrition Education

AUDREY TITTLE CROSS, J.D., M.P.H.
Nutrition Consultant
New York, New York

Address correspondence to Audrey Tittle Cross, J.D., 259 Sunset Ave., Englewood, New Jersey 07631.

ABSTRACT

The electronic era is upon us. Approximately seven million homes today have television sets which the average American spends about six hours daily watching. Over 300,000 computers for home use were purchased in 1983, and the number is rapidly increasing. Interactive television-computer programs are also on the rise.

Simultaneously, mushrooming interest in health, fitness, and diet has spawned bestseller books, a cadre of new magazines, health spas, and fitness wear and gear.

As a medium, television has responded slowly to the health craze. Television decision-makers at the national level view nutrition and health topics as limited in entertainment and commercial value.

Yet within local areas and in the near future through cable television, opportunities exist for dietitians and nutritionists to use television as an efficient and effective tool to reach the public. The spread of interactive television-computer programs also offers new opportunities for nutrition education.

Basic information on how to find a forum, prepare proposal presentations for segment concepts, determine production costs, and work with television personnel is outlined in the article.

INTRODUCTION

Food and nutrition are among the "hottest" areas of consumer interest today; and television is our most widespread communications medium. Yet only recently have the two begun to meet. What potential exists for introducing nutrition subjects on network and cable television? What do nutritionists need to know about the mechanics, operations, and economics of television to succeed in having nutrition messages aired? What future potential exists for use of this medium to reach the public with our messages?

252

AWARENESS AROUSED

Evidence of Interest

Public interest in health, fitness, and nutrition have grown astronomically over the past 10 years. Americans today believe, right or wrong, that fitness can meet a multitude of desires—to be young, rejuvenated, healthy, and attractive. Interest in food and nutrition issues has paralleled the increased interest in fitness, as has interest in gourmet cooking.

Surveys done by Yankelovich, Skelley and White, *Consumer Reports,* Gallup polls, *Self Magazine*'s Trends reports, and the Food Marketing Institute indicate that interest in nutrition is rising steadily and that nutrition considerations today are as important as food price in influencing food choice.

Persuasive evidence outside of surveys also points to the growing interest in nutrition, fitness, and health issues. For the past five years, no fewer than three books on diet, fitness, or health have consistently appeared on the *New York Times* weekly ten bestseller list. Several of these books, *Jane Brody's Nutrition Book,* Richard Simmons' *Never Say Diet, Beverly Hills Diet* by Judith Mazell, and *Life Extension* by Pearson and Shaw, have remained in the top ten at least six months or longer.

Magazines have also joined the movement. The last five years have seen the birth of a number of narrow audience magazines targeted exclusively to interest in health, diet, and fitness. *Shape, Fit, American Health, Muscle and Fitness, Bicycling, Self,* and *Runner's World,* to name a few, all carry regular features on food, diet, and nutrition. Until the debut of these magazines, only a small number of magazines that were sold in health food stores addressed these topics. The new genre of magazines is sold at grocery checkouts, at newsstands, and by subscription.

Magazines that traditionally wrote only recipes and articles on dieting have also altered their focus, no longer limiting articles to how to baste your turkey or your face. Today magazines like *Vogue, Good Housekeeping,* and *Harper's Bazaar* report breaking nutrition research news, in-depth analysis of current diet crazes, technical reports on food issues, and information on diet—disease interactions.

The Exercise Craze

There has also been an explosion of interest in exercise and fitness activities. The YMCA of the United States reports a national growth of 54% in family memberships between 1977 and 1982.

Until a few years ago, the "Y" and health spas like Venus spas and Jack LaLanne's centers dominated what little interest there was in exercise, body building, and fitness. Today their business is both expanding and meeting fierce competition from newcomers like Jane Fonda's Workouts, Nicholas Nautilus system centers, Richard Simmons' new exercise centers, and numerous other weight-lifting, body-building, sports, cardiovascular fitness, health, and exercise centers.

At one time Jack LaLanne was also our only television exercise personality, promising a marvelous musculature like his if you joined him in stretching and bending. Today's fitness guru, Richard Simmons, a small, impish, and energetic personality, offers exercise as the "feel good" alternative rather than as a road to a statuesque physique. His banter about food, diet, and exercise consistently nudges the Phil Donahue show (a talk show with diverse, interesting, and controversial guests) for the Neilsen ratings as the most popular morning television show.

For those who leave home before Simmons airs, there are several other television exercise options airing between 5:30 and 7:00 P.M. before the local and national morning news shows. "Morning Stretch," "20 Minute Workout," "Lilia's Yoga and You," and other local station variations on these network workouts. Alternatively we can catch early morning tips on health from "Health Field." Unfortunately, the nutritional information periodically included on these shows is often inaccurate and incomplete.

Food and Nutrition News

Those who flip on their television just in time to catch their favorite blond, Jane Pauley on the "Today Show," Diane Sawyer on "CBS Morning News," or Joan Lundgren on "Good Morning America," will also get consumer, health, nutrition, and fitness advice. Dr. Art Ulene, Tim Johnson, Frank Field, and other regulars on these shows report the latest news on everything from herpes to tennis elbow and bone meal.

While Richard Simmons' is the only network show devoted exclusively to fitness and health, there is a cable station that offers health features and programming. In early 1984, USA's Daytime, with programming for women viewers, merged with Cable Health Network, which had offered 24 hours of straight health programming. The new network, Lifetime, will carry a mixed program format of health and women's issues.

The TV Cooks

The nature of television cooking shows has also changed with the times. James Beard debuted as the first TV chef in 1946. He was followed in the 1960s by the popular Graham Kerr, "The Galloping Gourmet," and by Julia Child, the famed "French Chef." Ms. Child, who has received Emmy and Peabody awards, is still seen on ABC's "Good Morning America" and in her own syndicated show sold nationally to independent stations.

"PM Magazine's" Chef Tell is seen nationally by over 12 million viewers, and PBS airs seven segments on cooking, including "Slim Gourmet" and "Eat Well, Be Well," a segment sponsored by the Metropolitan Life Insurance Company. The very popular "Greengrocer," Joe Carcione, appears on newscasts to over 16 million viewers, offering tips on the selection of fresh produce. Cooking shows on several local stations have come and gone, as have cooking segments within variety shows such as "The Dinah Show."

Cooking style in these shows has changed significantly since James Beard and Julia Child first gave instructions for making Hollandaise Sauce and Baked Alaska. Many popular chefs have gone on diets to reduce their weight, their use of salt and fat, or both, and have published popular cookbooks filled with their new fat-free philosophies. As a consequence, today's TV recipes are simpler, require less time and skill in the kitchen, and often contain less fat, sugar, and salt than was once characteristic.

Approximately 70,000,000 homes have television sets. The average American watches television for 6 hours daily. Consumer interest in diet, nutrition, and fitness topics is clearly high. Just what does one need to know to either "break into TV" or to introduce nutrition topics into existing programs?

INDUSTRY STRUCTURE

The Networks

Television programming is provided by commercial, commercial-free, and cable companies. The major companies which dominate the airways are: National Broadcasting Corporation (NBC), Columbia Broadcasting Systems (CBS), and American Broadcasting Corporation (ABC), all headquartered in New York City. Between them they tie up almost 50% of all television airtime. They are commercial television, supported by companies who pay to have their advertisements on the air.

Commercial-free television, the Public Broadcasting Service (PBS), is supported by federal funds, contributions from private foundations, and donations from corporations and individuals. Advertising is specifically prohibited. However, when a petroleum company funds a major production for PBS, mention is usually made of the fact in the credits.

Cable television is pay TV. A monthly access fee is paid to receive programming transmitted by cable. It is predicted that 90% of all homes will have cable access by the year 1990. Cable is not commercial-free, though currently because fewer viewers use cable, commercial sponsorship has not reached the level existing for commercial television. Among the most widely distributed cable companies are Cable News Network (CNN), Daytime (owned by ABC/Hearst), and Music Television (MTV).

A network generally owns and operates several stations and also has station affiliates which air the same programs at the same time of day as if they were network owned and operated. Thus, NBC broadcasts the "Today Show" at 7 A.M. in each time zone across the nation on its wholly owned and operated stations and its affiliates as well. Similarly, CBS and its affiliates telecast "Magnum, P.I." at 8 P.M. on Thursdays across the nation.

Independently owned and operated stations for the most part do not air network-produced programming. Independents include stations such as KBHK, San Francisco; WHFT, Miami; and KMSP, Minneapolis. Generally the number of viewers watching these stations at any one time is significantly lower than the number simultaneously watching any one of the networks in the same city.

Programming

Because prime-time programming is so important to a network's ratings, power, and prestige, limited leeway exists for local decisionmaking by either the network station or its affiliates. Decisions affecting this time are made at headquarters by the directors of the programming departments (news, entertainment, special events, sports, etc.) and the director of business affairs. Jointly they are responsible for selecting programs that will competitively draw viewers from simultaneously aired programs on other networks and thereby attract substantial advertisment revenues to their stations.

Networks produce their own news segments, sports, special programming (such as movies produced for television or documentaries on personalities or events), and some game and talk shows.

These programs must be aired by an affiliate or network station during what is called weekday "network" time. This is from 7:00 A.M.

until 9:00 A.M.; from 10:00 A.M. (11:00 A.M. for ABC) until 4:30 P.M.; for a half-hour at either 6:30 or 7:00 P.M. for the evening network news; from 8:00 P.M. until 11:00 P.M.; and if the station chooses to air "Wide World of Entertainment," "Tonight Show" or "Late Movies," until those segments end.

In the remaining time, the stations can air programs of their choice: from sign-on until 7:00 A.M., between 9:00 A.M. and 10:00 A.M., from 4:30 P.M. to 8:00 P.M., and from 11:00 P.M. to sign-off. Because of expanded sports coverage and programming on weekends, stations have fewer and fewer weekend hours available for their own programming.

Time slots not dominated by the networks are filled with either locally produced programming or with syndicated shows purchased from outside producers. A station will commonly run its own local news show in the pre-network slot. For example, "Mornings at Five" on Nashville's NBC affiliate, WTVF, or "Good Morning from Memphis" on ABC's WREG.

The mid-morning slot may be filled with a locally produced talk show, such as the "Bob Braun Show" on WLWT (NBC) in Cincinnati or "Katherine's Show" on KPRC (NBC) in Houston, or with a syndicated game show. The early evening slots are commonly filled with locally produced news or news-type shows, for example, "Stone at Five" on KPRC, Houston, and "Layman and Company" on KXAS (NBC) in Dallas, or with syndicated shows like "I Love Lucy." Again, after 11:00 P.M. stations may air their own shows, "All Night Alive" on KOA (NBC), Denver, or syndicated movies or reruns.

Weekend time is often filled with cartoons, local community billboard shows featuring local issues and leaders as guests, news, reruns of movies and old television serial shows, and network-programmed sports packages.

Independent stations, which are not network owned or affiliated, have only station time and exercise complete discretion over programming. Because of the high cost of quality program production, these stations often purchase a great deal of programming from independent syndicators rather than fund original programming.

In the early days of television, very few programs were made specifically for syndicated sales. "Jack LaLanne" was one of the few. Today a large number of shows is either independently syndicated or syndicated by a network. The "Richard Simmons Show" is privately syndicated while "PM Magazine" (also called "Evening Magazine") is produced and syndicated by Westinghouse Broadcasting. Because these are not network exclusive shows, they can be sold to network stations, network affiliates, and to independent stations. For example, the "Mike Douglas Show" is telecast on more than 200 stations.

Cost of Production

The cost to produce a show from inception to airing is difficult to estimate. An hour-long prime-time dramatic show can cost from $275,000 to $300,000, a variety show from $200,000 to $300,000. These are costs per episode!

At one time, advertising agencies produced shows for either groups or individual commercial sponsors. The "Colgate Comedy Hour" and "Kraft Theatre" were examples. The "Galloping Gourmet" was produced by Young and Rubicam, an advertising agency, as a vehicle to advertise the various food and household products of its clients.

Today, programs are not owned or produced by a single advertising agency or a single commercial sponsor. Neither do sponsors exercise any direct control over program format or content. Their sole option is to withdraw commercial sponsorship from a program if they find its contents to be objectionable or to conflict with sales promotion goals. Notwithstanding that direct control over program content is not exercised, it is not surprising that producers are "sensitive" to the needs of their sponsors and generally will not include program content which "bites the hand that feeds it."

Commercial time is sold in units of 30, 45, 60, and 90 seconds. The cost to purchase a unit depends upon the number of viewers who are expected to be watching when the commercial is aired. Thus, 60 seconds can cost as little as $1000 during the early evening news segment of an independent station to as much as $60,000 for a minute on the popular "Tonight Show."

The Ratings

To the advertiser who wants to invest money in mass media marketing, the critical question is, how many people can be reached per dollar spent? There are no ticket receipts to tell you how many people watched the "Saturday Night Movies."

The authority on who is watching what and when is the A.C. Nielsen company which publishes the *Nielsen Television Index*, called the "Nielsen ratings." The ratings are based on viewing information collected every 15 minutes by mechanical recording devices attached to televisions in 1700 sample households around the country.

Ratings predict the percentage of total televisions available (70,000,000) which tuned to a program. A rating of 10 indicates that 10% of those available, approximately 7 million television sets, turned on the program. Nielsen estimates that each television is viewed by 2.2 people; thus, over 15 million people watched the program.

The data are reported in several forms, the most important of which are the "nationals," reported every other week, and the "sweeps," reported in February, May, and November. The sweeps are conducted by asking a sample of households to keep a diary of its viewing for one week. Samples are taken so that ratings can be reported for each individual station in the country.

Ratings are used by the networks to determine which shows will be continued or canceled. They are used by advertisers to decide whether and how much they will pay for a commercial time slot during any given program.

ACCESSING THE AIR

The Opportunities

Clearly, health, nutrition, and fitness are issues of current popular interest. So much so that the interest has spawned bestselling books, magazines devoted exclusively to fitness topics, and a cable television station featuring only health and fitness programming.

For those interested in using television as a vehicle for reaching mass populations with nutrition messages, what opportunities exist or could be developed?

Realistically, the networks are not the place to look for air time. While there is increasing public interest in nutrition, it is still considered to be a "serious" topic that should be addressed by the "experts" and then only periodically on news or magazine format shows (such as "Hour Magazine"). It is not believed that the field has significant "entertainment" value, nor that the degree of public interest is wide enough to merit frequent or regular network time. It is felt that what public interest there is, is either met by other media forms (narrow-market magazines) or can be served by periodic inclusion of an "expert" on the news.

Even cooking shows are not highly rated. Only one television cook, Julia Child, currently has a financially successful show, and it is underwritten and produced by PBS rather than a commercial network. Nor does it air during "network" time on the affiliates that have purchased the show.

Another issue that deters production of a nutrition/food show is commercial sponsorship. The most probable sponsors are food product manufacturers. Sponsorship of a nutrition show would suggest food product endorsement by the show. Most nutritionists do not want to endorse products. Neither would most nutritionists consent to censure of program content by a sponsor to ensure lack of conflict with the sponsor's proprietary interests. Conversely, most sponsors would not want to fund programming in which there was risk that comments made on the show might result in commercial damage.

If no one will sponsor or air a half-hour nutrition show, and if "Good Morning America" and "Phil Donahue" are only interested in infrequent appearances by luminaries such as Mark Hegsted, Ph.D., Harvard University, or Myron Winick, M.D., director of the Human Nutrition Institute at Columbia University, what is left?

Finding a Forum

While opportunities are few, they do exist. Shows of lesser status, for example, "Good Morning New York" in Manhattan and "Good Morning" in San Francisco, will book appearances by "lesser" experts such as faculty from local colleges, clinical dietitians from major local hospitals, heads of home economics programs in extension offices, or home economists working with food trade associations. With the proper presentation, they might also be convinced to include a regular segment on food and nutrition in their show.

Local news shows, the noon or early evening news, might accept regular appearances to give diet tips, food and consumer information on purchasing, label reading, and so forth, or interpretation of recent research findings. These are usually 30- to 90-second spots.

Locally hosted talk or variety shows offer the potential for longer segments. Appearances might be made for in-depth discussions of current nutrition or diet issues such as anorexia, the effects of color and flavor additives on behavior, or alcohol and pregnancy. Demonstrations are popular on this type of show—how to read a vitamin supplement label, how to use whole grains in menu planning, how to prepare baby foods at home, and so on.

While it is obviously much more feasible to initiate appearances or segments within an existing show than it is to create a new show, it is not impossible. A local, independently owned station or a cable station serving a local area is more likely to consider a new show than is a network station or affiliate. They have more time available for locally produced programming than do networks or affiliates. The cost of production for independent station shows is also considerably lower than for networks. Local sponsors such as bakeries, food processors, or local grocery chains might be enlisted to fund production costs and purchase commercial time on a show.

Presentations

Whether the show is "Good Morning America" or "Greetings to Gary, Indiana," a "handle" is needed to interest the producer in devoting air time to nutrition. A "handle" is a story line, a pitch, a catchy, controversial, or even corny presentation of an idea. The most important criterion is that it must be able to get and keep the attention of the viewers.

Viewers are *not* interested in stories that are discouraging, disgusting, dry and boring, old news which they either know already or have heard too many times before, or which makes them feel guilty, stupid, or failing. They do not want lectures, long-winded answers to simple questions, nor threats about negative consequences if they choose to disregard the advice given.

Television is an entertainment medium, and above all, viewers are interested in being entertained. They want whatever information that is given to them to be funny, upbeat, likeable, easy to do, different, a little naughty, and fast. If the answer takes longer than 30 seconds, they are not interested. They reason that if it takes so long to explain, it must be difficult. And they are not interested in difficulty. They want easy, happy, quick results, not drudgery.

Those presenting an idea for either an appearance on a show or a regular segment on a show should be cognizant of these sentiments. Producers are extremely sensitive to viewer preference, ratings, and sponsor reactions.

A proposal to appear as a guest on a show or to start a regular segment on the show is made to the producer of the show. A proposal to initiate a new show (e.g., a 30-minute food and nutrition program) is made to the station producer. Make an inquiry phone call to the producer to see if any thread of interest exists. Then develop a written presentation of the idea. Whatever the content of the idea (diet and cancer, brain and mood food, for example) keep the presentation simple, light, and punchy. Remember these are entertainment people. They are *not* academicians, health service administrators, or county agents. This is show time!

Producers are busy people. Your presentation should be simple, easy to read (lots of white space on the page), and should get to the point quickly. On the first page give your name and the phone number at which you can be reached (or rejected). Then briefly summarize your concept and why you should do the appearance.

If the presentation is to create a show, include a minute-by-minute format outline of the show, list types of props or staging required, names of potential guests, on-location filming, if any, and so on. State the estimated cost of production and who will sponsor these costs. If possible, arrange to have production done by a company already known to the station producer. This will lend credibility to it.

If you have appeared on television before, send along a video tape of your appearance. If not, enclose a black and white glossy photo. Be honest with yourself about your physical appearance. No matter how pertinent, current, or cleverly presented, diet advice from an overweight person is not believable. In television, one picture is truly worth a thousand words.

When the producer has had a few days to look at your proposal, give them a call. Do not wait for a written response. Producers are often too busy for such formalities. Ask for an appointment to discuss your proposal or for a date for an appearance on the show.

Be flexible. The producer may like your idea in part but not in whole. Accept and use their criticisms. This is their business. If the producer says the topic is only worth 45 seconds instead of the 6 minutes which you prepared, condense it. State the salient points and forget the fluff.

Production

Once your concept or show is ready for shooting, you will meet several other key television personnel. The first will probably be the show's writer. The writer will prepare the introduction and questions that the host or hostess of the show will use during your appearance.

The set, the location where the television show is made, is supervised by the director. The director decides camera angles, lighting, timing, and if the show is taped instead of live, whether or not to reshoot, that is, to repeat, a segment. In television, the director may also be the producer or may be called an associate producer.

When appearing on a live show, there will be no opportunity for correction of mistakes. Therefore, practice answering questions that you expect to be asked. Practice quickly condensing an answer in case the director begins signaling that it is time to break for a commercial or to move on to the next segment of the show.

If the show is taped for airing at a later date, you may or may not have the opportunity to reshoot a "flub." If you are very concerned about a statement made, ask the director if it is possible to retake the answer. This often is possible when taping.

While only one or two people may be seen on camera, numerous people support production of a show. Camera operators, lighting experts, make-up artists, set designers, timers, floor director, word monitor operators, and others, do their part to get a show to the air.

And tucked away in the control room are editors, sound and color mixing experts, electronic technicians and others blending together the various elements of the show and feeding them to the airways.

Making It

Succeeding in this medium is a precarious proposition at best. Few survive the fickle attention span of viewers. This season's most popular sitcom (situation comedy) may hold its own in the ratings for two sweeps, only to fall short in the third and be cancelled. Even extremely popular series ("Gunsmoke" and "Hogan's Heroes") were eventually canceled.

Fortunately, predictions for the future include uses of television other than as an entertainment medium. It is believed, and there is already rapid movement in this direction, that television will be used extensively in classrooms, clinics, and marketplaces to provide information and education in much the same way teachers, libraries, and other information resources do today.

The rapid expansion of computers in these same settings will allow for interactive learning through television-computer hookups. Kaiser-Permanente Medical Group in Oakland, California has pioneered in this area, providing a multimedia health education center where patients can seek information on their own about their diagnosis and treatment, using film, audio and video tapes, and computerized learning programs. A system called QUBE-TV, being tested in Columbus, Ohio and several other cities, allows viewers to interact with their television sets, promising to bring interactive learning directly to the home.

The tools which nutritionists, home economists, and dietitians use today to communicate information about food and nutrition will one day be replaced by electronic media. Our pamphlets will be available for call-up on a computer screen. Our classes, whether for diabetics, pregnant or nursing mothers, or preschoolers, will be aired regularly on channels devoted to health and fitness concerns. Viewers will be able to type questions to us via computer just as live audiences today ask questions of talk show guests.

Until the electronic age arrives, there are opportunities to present our messages on local news and talk shows as a guest, whether frequent or infrequent. There are opportunities to be included as a regular segment in ongoing programs such as local variety and talk shows. Where local independent and cable stations exist, there are opportunities to produce a regular weekly show on food and nutrition issues.

The competition for these opportunities is fierce. In television, almost as in no other arena, time is money. Access to airtime is guarded cautiously by those who are accountable for its monetary success. The opportunities that exist will not come knocking on your door. It is you who must go door to door, knocking and seeking to convince the powers that be that nutrition is marketable.

INDEX

265